Finding X

One Family's Solution to Obsessive Compulsive Disorder

Also by Ray St. John

The Ray of Hope: A Teenager's Fight Against Obsessive Compulsive Disorder

Finding X

One Family's Solution to Obsessive Compulsive Disorder

Joni St. John

Ray St. John

Vermilion Press - 2013

Vermilion Press
8008 E. 2600 N. Rd
Manville, IL 61319

Vermilionpress@gmail.com

Cover photograph by: H. Tak Cheung

Finding X: One Family's Solution to Obsessive Compulsive Disorder/ Joni St. John and Ray St. John

ISBN: 978-1-4675-6762-6

Library of Congress Control Number: 2013935015

First Printing, 2013

In loving memory of our mother, grandmother, and fellow sufferer of OCD

Frieda St. John

Contents

Part IV – Additional Ideas for Treating OCD

Part V – Additional Issues on OCD

Our Purpose For This Book

Here is yet another book on obsessive compulsive disorder (OCD). Sorry. We couldn't help writing it; it just slipped out. With the hundreds of OCD books already written it's hard to imagine that there would be anything for us to add. In fact, we are even responsible for one of those books (*The Ray of Hope: A Teenager's Fight Against Obsessive Compulsive Disorder*); so why did we keep going and add even more of our OCD story to the pile? The short answer to this question is simply this: We wanted to help our fellow sufferers of OCD who continue to struggle with it. Even with all the information that is currently available on OCD, many people still suffer terribly. We never have to look far before we see the damage OCD continues to make. It still cripples lives, both young and old, because many who have it go untreated, receive inappropriate care, or only get partial treatment.

There are medications that are used to help those who have OCD and a therapeutic approach that has been proven to help alleviate its symptoms, but yet OCD stubbornly continues to affect many people. Why this happens isn't clear, but we suspect that several factors are involved, such as misdiagnosis of OCD, miserable side effects from the medications used to treat OCD, stigma surrounding mental health disorders, mental health professionals who remain ignorant of the current recommended treatment for OCD, and the pain that is often involved even when the right treatment is applied. With all these factors working against us, it's a miracle that anyone with OCD can find the path to good mental health.

But, many of us do. That is, we have found our way out of OCD and into a better world. How we do it, however, often results not from following a well-defined map but from blazing our own trail. With only a few, general directions, we pick our way along dark and winding paths until we either reach our destination or decide to turn back and find another way. This journey is not for the fainthearted or the uncommitted. We wish we could say otherwise, that once someone with OCD gets the right diagnosis and finds their way to a well-trained mental health professional that all they have to do is sit back and wait for the magic to happen. Sadly, it doesn't happen this way. Dealing with a mental illness is nothing like receiving treatment for many physical illnesses where improvement, or even a cure, often entails just a few intravenous injections or a surgical procedure.

Because recovery from OCD forces us to walk a twisted and individual path, it's important that each of us who need to take this journey gather up as many tools and maps as we can before starting out. This is where we hope our book can help. In it, we show the path we took to get out of our own OCD hell. We know that our path will not be exactly like the one everyone else needs to take, but we suspect that, in many ways, it will be similar. After all, we are all starting from a similar place (OCD) and trying to reach the same destination (mental health). There are bound to be paths we share, markers we recognize, and barriers we all have to overcome as we make this journey.

We wish this book could do more than what it does. We would love to be the ones to write the "Manual in Curing OCD," the one book that describes the step-by-step process that is guaranteed to cure all who have OCD of their affliction. Truth is, I doubt that such a book will ever be written. I also doubt that a pill will be formulated that controls all symptoms of OCD or that a surgical procedure will be developed that erases all aberrant brain pathways that cause OCD. OCD is too diverse, acts so differently in each one it touches, and disguises itself so well that I can't imagine that only one intervention could ever help all those who have OCD.

Overcoming OCD is similar to solving any other complicated problem. There is the goal (eg, navigating our way through school, finding someone to share our lives with, achieving and maintaining our financial health, or in our case, obtaining and maintaining mental health) and there are the variables we have to identify and manage (eg, what school to go to, what job to try for, where to live, or what medication or therapist to try) in order to achieve our goals. In other words, we can think of our goal as an "X" to solve (like in a mathematical problem) and the formula for solving it as consisting of the many variables. With OCD, we all share the goal of achieving mental health but differ in some of the variables we need to manage to get there. What we hope to accomplish with this book is to help those who are struggling with their OCD find and manage some of the many variables they need. We hope that by showing how we solved our "X" that others will also find their way to mental health.

But before we get too far, let us introduce ourselves. My son, Ray, is the one whose story you will hear about the most. His OCD was identified the earliest in life and because of that, he has done well. He is currently in college and has managed his OCD to the point where it rarely bothers him and when it does, it's quickly stamped out. I have never been officially diagnosed with OCD but can definitely see its hand in my life. I can identify many episodes where OCD was in charge, even though I wasn't aware that what I was experiencing even had a name. Today, I have only minimal OCD symptoms and in fact, have not had any major OCD flare-ups for many years. Overall, I have done fairly well in life; I got through medical school and was a pediatrician in a small community until Ray's OCD threatened to take over his life. At that time, I stepped back from my career to help him. Even though it's our voices, mine and Ray's, that are heard in this book, we have also added the story of a third family member who was affected by OCD: My mother. Like me, she was never officially diagnosed with OCD, but there is no doubt that she had it. In fact, I am convinced that OCD was partially responsible for her early death.

In this book, it's my voice that is louder and more militant than Ray's. To his credit, Ray has decided that he wants to reach beyond his OCD and go on, whereas I sometimes get mired in the past. Because of this tendency, however, I remember more of our OCD stories than what Ray does and can reveal more about what we went through. I am also much more protective of our story. Where others probably would let the past go, especially those parts where difficulties and pain are concerned, I often keep it alive. I do this because we need to remember what we used to beat back OCD and to keep those tools readily available for the time when OCD tries to come back. I remember so that I can stay ready.

The OCD stories and ideas in this book are ours; no one else has touched them (no reviewers, editors, or publishers). We wrote, edited, and then published this book on our own. We did this because we didn't want any filters between us and our readers and wanted to preserve the main purpose of this book, which is simply this: Two people describing their experiences with OCD in the hope that their stories can help others who have OCD. We worried that if we listened to the opinions of those who hadn't personally experienced OCD, our book might lose some of its authenticity and its ability to help. Maybe a professional editor would have made this book easier to read or more entertaining, but at the same time, they may have changed it in many unhelpful ways.

A final note: We encourage anyone who is reading this book to skip around and pick out those sections that are most useful to them. We have written this book in such a way so that individual sections can stand alone. If, for example, you're not quite sure of our credentials in talking about OCD, then please read about our OCD stories so that you are reassured that we genuinely have OCD. If, however, you want to know how we dealt with OCD, then go straight to the sections where we describe the therapy we used. Even though we hope that the entire book is useful, we understand if some readers only read parts of it. We certainly don't want to waste anyone's time, especially with regards to dealing with OCD. So, our advice is simply to pick and choose whatever sections you think might help.

Ray also hopes that what we have written helps those who continue to struggle with OCD. He knows all too well what OCD can do and the havoc it can cause.

ΔΔΔΔ

Because of OCD, years of my life have gone by, without a trace and with barely even one happy memory that can be drawn from them. It almost feels like I really should be sixteen right now instead of nineteen because I missed out on discoveries and friendships I could have made, people whom I could have been inspired by, and great experiences that could have shaped who I am. Nothing fills those few years but wasted time and regret, and this is not a fate I want anyone to share. I want people to read this book and heed my words so that they can see the absurdity in their OCD as I see it now and get back to their lives. I want to help others with OCD to fully become the people they can be.

During my freshman and sophomore years of high school I had no friends. I was undoubtedly, the least social person in my class, as I could barely hold a conversation with anyone about anything. I had no particular skills or interests that could be discussed, and my sense of humor was nonexistent. I'm sure that many others in my class looked at me and felt a sort of pity and disdain; they knew that I had struggles, but they had no intention or motivation to help me out of that gutter. Therefore, I never made any real friends, and school became a place of pure anxiety. In hindsight, my lack of sociality was a nasty side effect of having OCD. Even if someone would reach out to me and try to talk to me, I would not have any room in my brain to formulate a response because of countless OCD thoughts that were racing through my head. I remember one particular example when a girl asked me where I had gone to middle school. While my mind was reaching for a response, I immediately felt guilty for talking to a girl (my OCD was focusing on sexual matters at that time), and all recollection that she had asked me a question faded. Not only was I seen as weird for not answering her question, I seemed stupid.

I can remember countless other examples of awkward situations, and I hate my OCD because of the way it forced me to interact with others. It took me years to get to a level of sociality that was acceptable, and because of my OCD, I have missed out on so many fun experiences with life. Talking with others, giving to them, and taking from them are truly the interactions that make us happy as human beings. OCD took years of that away from me. This is the one thing I hate OCD the most for.

I know that there are many others who now suffer from OCD in the same way I did. At one time, OCD thoughts flooded my conscious mind every second of the day, and my development as a person suffered because of it. Hopefully, through my experiences and this book, others can take my advice and apply it and in doing so, destroy their OCD like the plague it is.

Part I - Our OCD stories

Introduction to Our OCD Stories

There are only a few things in life of which we all are certain, such as the effects of gravity, the forward progression of time, and the inevitability of death. But, we also carry with us through our lives personal certainties that are not universal. For me, there is one certainty that few others even think about let alone share: My absolute hatred of OCD. I hate OCD with all my being and at times, I have even feared what that hatred might spur me to do. As I have gotten older, however, and as OCD has lessened its effects on me, I have tempered that hatred so it's not so close to the surface; I no longer base my life or my decisions on OCD and have found a healthier and more productive way to live. What I can also say, however, is that my hatred of OCD is still very much alive and if given the right chance, may spring back to life and take control.

It's understandable if other sufferers of OCD don't share my hatred of it. Maybe their case was mild, only slightly affecting their lives and easily eradicated once it was identified. Maybe their OCD was incorporated into their lives and used as a positive force for good. I have heard several OCD advocates say that OCD made them into who they are, that they wouldn't change their lives, or that they credit OCD for some of the good that they have experienced. Not me. This will never be my view on OCD.

There are many who might think that my hatred of OCD is strange and counterproductive and that I should find ways to make peace with its presence in this world. Why not just accept that OCD exists and allow it to find its place in the lives of those it afflicts? Why not accept that some of us will always have OCD and find ways to use it in a good way? There are times when I considered stopping my anti-OCD militancy and wondered if I could form a détente with OCD. But then, memories of what OCD did to me

16

and my family would surface, and I knew that compromise was impossible. In our family, OCD has caused early death, disability, and has threatened our futures. For us, living with OCD is like having our own personal terrorist who lives in our home, takes our resources, threatens us with terrible consequences if we don't do what he says, and refuses all attempts to ouster him. Who wouldn't hate such a terrorist? Who wouldn't lay down their own life in the attempt to retake the life of a loved one who had been taken by such a terrorist?

In our family, there are three of us who have dealt with OCD. My son, Ray, whose experience is laid bare in this book, is the only one who has been officially diagnosed with OCD by a mental health professional. The other two of us, my mother and I, have never been diagnosed with OCD but have graced the offices of several psychiatrists where we received diagnoses such as general anxiety disorder (GAD) and dysthymia. But when a closer look is taken at our symptoms, it's obvious that OCD has had a hand in hurting us. Why our psychiatrists chose other diagnoses, instead of OCD, isn't clear. In my case, I think it was because OCD had beaten me down and had caused me to take so many wrong turns in life that I had become too depressed to really function anymore. I acted and looked more like someone who has depression than someone who has OCD. As for my mother, it was most likely a case of semi-misdiagnosis (as GAD). Her psychiatrist was close in that GAD and OCD can look a lot alike; he just hadn't spent the time to look closer at my mother's symptoms and see the OCD.

Grandma's OCD Story

Of the three of us, my mother's (Ray's grandma) OCD story is the most incomplete. She died, at age sixty-one, long before Ray's OCD showed itself and before it had occurred to me that OCD was a large part of my thinking. I am certain, however, that Grandma's brain had been affected by OCD and that her life would have been more complete if it had been realized and treated. The clearest example of her OCD occurred about a year before her death when she suddenly became obsessed about my father and the possibility that he might be hurt. She wasn't worried about all types of injuries, however, but one specific and highly unusual one: She obsessed over my father getting struck by lightning. To help alleviate her fears, she would compulsively do several things, such as following my father around to reassure herself that he was safe, repeatedly scan the sky for black clouds so that she was certain that no storms were impending, or ask whoever was physically closest to her if they thought my father was all right (ie, seeking reassurance). My father didn't know what to do, so he did what most would do in these types of situations. He tried to reassure her that he was fine, had always been fine with regards to weather-related incidents, and couldn't possibly think of any situation where his safety would be threatened by weather. He repeatedly told her that he was not careless, that he had enough sense to get to shelter when storms hit, and that all of her fears were nonsense. Words such as these, even though helpful for garden-variety worries, only served to feed Grandma's OCD, and it continued to grow.

Why Grandma's OCD latched onto lightning and its exceedingly rare lethality will never be clear to us. But, we also know that it's not important to figure out. OCD latches onto the nearest fear it can find, not caring how rare, obtuse, or fantastical that fear may be. Our best guess as to why lightning figured in Grandma's OCD was because

18

she had lived for most of her life on a farm, a place where weather is figured into many decisions. Perhaps somewhere in her memory was stored a time when someone mentioned how bad or dangerous a particular storm was and how they needed to be careful. Just a few, seemingly innocuous words would be enough for OCD to find a foothold.

Grandma's OCD finally got the best of my father, and he had her admitted to our local hospital where she underwent a barrage of tests, none of which helped explain her symptoms. Since our community was too small to support any behavioral health services, we had to find help elsewhere and finally located a psychiatrist who would see her. After a short visit, he declared that she had general anxiety disorder and prescribed an antidepressant, imipramine (this was shortly before Prozac and the other, newer antidepressants had become widely available). No other therapy was suggested, and we were too ignorant at the time to ask for additional help, such as a therapist for Grandma to talk to. With no other viable ideas, Grandma decided to take the imipramine and hope that it would help quell her fears and allow her to return to normal. What happened next, however, was something we have never quite understood: Grandma's OCD suddenly disappeared.

Unfortunately, the disappearance of Grandma's OCD coincided with a physical disaster: Her heart failed. One day she suddenly noticed that her feet were swollen and that her breathing felt more difficult. Her doctor quickly diagnosed heart failure, admitted her to the local hospital, but then transported her to a larger, better equipped hospital that was located a couple of hours away. Somewhere during that transport her OCD melted away, but because we were all so worried about her heart, it took us several hours to realize the change. We were sitting by her bedside waiting for any number of things to happen, doctors to show up, orderlies to take her for tests, or nurses to come with medications to administer, when it occurred to us that she hadn't mentioned her worries about my father getting struck by lightning. It had been a relentless mantra of hers for months and now there was a silence. In fact, she even looked happy. Here she was in a large, chaotic hospital, not knowing what was to happen with her heart or if she might have to undergo some risky surgery, and she looked happier than she had for months. It was like someone had waved a magic wand and poof, the OCD was gone.

We were flabbergasted but cautiously hopeful that her mind had somehow healed itself. No one really credited the imipramine for helping her OCD; there hadn't been enough time for it to have reached therapeutic levels. In fact, one doctor even suggested that the imipramine had somehow pushed her heart into failure. The older antidepressants, such as imipramine and desipramine, are well known for their deleterious side effects, including ones that affect the heart, so it was entirely possible that the medication she was prescribed to help her brain had instead, pushed her heart into failure.

The doctors we asked were equally clueless as to why her OCD had magically disappeared (in fact, I doubted if any of them knew much about OCD). The only one who even ventured a guess was her cardiologist, who suggested that maybe she had felt panicky because of fluid that had accumulated in her lungs secondary to her heart failure. This fluid had caused her to feel short of breath, which she might have mistaken for her fears. Once the fluid had been removed via medications, then maybe, she no longer felt fearful. At the time, we thought this idea was plausible and accepted it. Nothing else had made any sense, so it seemed reasonable that her physical problems had contributed to her mental symptoms. We also readily accepted this explanation because it was comforting to do so. If her symptoms were related to a physical condition, then it meant that they could be more easily fixed.

Grandma's heart gave out for good about a year after her OCD episode had vanished. During that year, we saw no overt evidence of obsessions, and she never mentioned having any. She seemed happy, relaxed, and was enjoying life. We never again mentioned her fears mainly because we were afraid of triggering them again, like breathing life into a sleeping monster. In retrospect, I wished she had been asked to explain what had happened to her thinking during the time when her OCD was active. Maybe her experience would have helped me identify and deal with Ray's OCD when it stirred for the first time. With her experience in mind, maybe I could have recognized Ray's OCD quicker and not have wasted time hoping that it would go away. I would have been primed to fight if off instead of just letting it passively stroll into my home. But, we will never know. We chose not to talk about it, bring it out into the open where we could dissect it, figure it out, and prepare ourselves for the time when it might return. Which, of course, it did.

Because we never openly talked about Grandma's symptoms before her death, her entire OCD story has been lost. What is left are fragments of memories which I have tried to sew together into a coherent story that makes sense. Even though clear-cut OCD symptoms are not readily remembered by anyone who was close to Grandma, I am convinced that OCD was in control of her life for years, maybe even for most of her life. This conclusion is based on how most of my memories of her are accompanied by sadness and a resignation that my mother suffered in ways that other mothers didn't. Where other mothers were active in their kid's schools, held down jobs, planted huge gardens, or actively volunteered in the community, my mother did mainly one thing: She sat. There was one particular chair in our living room that was hers, and she could often be found sitting there, reading during the day or watching television in the evening. She never had any hobbies, many friends to call up or to do things with, or even any desire to change her situation. To her credit, she did try to fulfill her duties as a housewife and mother; she put meals on the table but rarely tried to cook new dishes or experiment with old ones; she cleaned the house on the occasion when it got so dirty that my father threatened to clean it if she didn't; and she attended my school functions. Sometimes, she would even spark to life a little and find somewhere for us to go, like a play, an open house, or a new restaurant. But mainly, she remained in her house and in her chair.

Grandma's shrunken world and how it came to be made sense to me after reading several books on OCD. Those who have OCD experience such intense anxiety that they will do anything to avoid whatever triggers that anxiety. If, for example, someone fears germs, then they will avoid places which they feel are contaminated, such as public restrooms or restaurants. And if left untreated, their OCD may eventually, cause them to avoid all contact with others or even result in them refusing to leave their germ-free home. Several people who have OCD have even gotten so bad that they no longer wear clothes, leave their beds, or talk to anyone. In Grandma's case, it was probably her anxiety that gradually resulted in her withdrawal from the world. What specifically she was anxious about, I don't know, but I do remember her becoming easily worried and expressing that worry. I even learned not to trigger her worries and for most of my childhood was very careful not to do or say anything that might upset her. I tried to be perfect for her, getting good grades, never arguing with her, staying home and not going out with peers, and not experimenting with all those things, such as alcohol or sexual matters, that most teenagers try to some extent. In this case, OCD not only shrunk her world but also mine.

Grandma's situation was complicated by another factor: Her obesity. Which came first, her mental issues or her obesity, isn't clear, but it's likely that her mental distress resulted in her overeating and in her inactivity, which then led to her obesity. In fact, it was this health condition with its accompanying hypertension and diabetes that caused her early death. She had neglected her health for so many years that eventually, her heart couldn't take the stress any longer and failed. It had tried to warn her on several occasions by having several, small heart attacks but even then, she failed to listen. When the cause of her death is closely examined, the following scenario seems most likely: Stress from OCD or another anxiety disorder came first, which she then attempted to alleviate by eating (eating has been shown to help with some anxiety). Because she was experiencing so much stress, the fat that resulted from her overeating was deposited in her abdomen instead of in other places, such as her thighs or buttocks (ie, she was more apple-shaped than pear-shaped). This is important because it's now well known that certain types of fat distribution are more highly associated with heart disease than others and that stress, via a complicated cascade of hormones, causes fat to accumulate in the more heart-damaging areas. In short, Grandma's OCD resulted in her eating her way into an early grave.

Where Grandma's OCD came from is not known; did it start with her or did she inherit it from her parents? Perhaps her mother or father also had symptoms but were so adept at hiding them that no one ever knew. Maybe their symptoms were such that they found ways to accommodate their obsessions into their daily lives. They were farmers, living most of their lives away from others and during a time when most farmers kept to themselves and when most women stayed in their homes. They also lived during the time when both men and women of the farming community had to work from sunup to sundown just to survive. In other words, maybe any OCD tendencies that they had were suppressed by their daily activities and never had a chance to gain a foothold. It is well known that OCD can flare during times when a mind is idle; in fact, one suggestion that is often found in OCD books is for those who have OCD to find ways to stay busy. Maybe for some, like my grandparents, their daily lives are forcibly so active that it protects them from certain mental disorders, such as OCD. But, we will never know whether they, or any of their ancestors, sparked the OCD that was to plague their descendants or whether it arose for the first time in Grandma.

My OCD Story

Next up in our family's OCD story is me. Like my mother, I have never been officially diagnosed with OCD. My own trip to the psychiatrist's office, at age forty-six, resulted in a diagnosis of dysthymia, a chronic, unrelenting, low-grade form of depression. How I ended up with dysthymia is unclear, but I am convinced that OCD had a hand in leading me there.

My first memories of having OCD-like thoughts occurred when I was about seven. And like in many cases, my "thoughts" arose quickly. I was in first grade doing what first graders normally do, but then one day, it all changed. Even now I can picture the moment when it happened and can bring up the same emotions that were felt during that moment. It was during recess, and I was playing with some classmates in the school gym. I had decided that it would be more fun to go back to the classroom with some friends and mess around there. Of course, we didn't have permission to do this, but being kids, we did it anyway. After returning to the gym, the teacher called me over and asked me where I had been. Instead of telling the truth, I lied. I said that I had been in the bathroom all the time and added something about having to go poop so that it would appear reasonable why so much time had passed. The teacher accepted my explanation and all seemed well for a while. Shortly, however, that one lie started haunting my thoughts. I couldn't let it go but turned it over and over again. It became stuck in an endless loop in my mind, and I spent hours worrying about it. My main concerns were that I was no longer a good kid and that if my parents knew about my lie, they would no longer love me and want me around. It's hard to remember how long I obsessed over this one lie because it happened so long ago, but I know that it lasted for several months. I remember feeling lonely, sad, and guilty. I even remember thinking that it wasn't fair that a kid like me had to deal with these feelings.

One day, relief from my obsessions suddenly happened. I don't remember how this day came about, but I decided to confess my terrible sin. I gathered up my courage, decided to face whatever might happen, and told my mother. I told her how I had lied to my teacher. I can still remember the feelings of relief that flooded through me when she didn't react. She smiled at me and told me not to worry because all kids make mistakes. I didn't tell her, however, how long I had been worrying and how much that worrying had taken away from me. I was so relieved that it didn't occur to me to tell her the whole story.

The relief I felt from that first confession was strong. It was like finally being released from prison and seeing the sunlight. But soon afterward, the worrying started up again. This time, however, I knew what to do to feel better: Confess my thoughts. I started on a marathon of confessions. I told my mother everything that I had ever done or thought that I felt was bad. If I wasn't sure if something was bad, I confessed it anyway just so I could feel the relief. Like an addict who craves their drug of choice, I craved those feelings of relief. Looking back, it's clear that it was OCD driving my thoughts and behavior, but at the time, we didn't know that anything was wrong. What my mother thought about my endless confessions we will never know. I have no memories of her asking me about my worries and why I felt so strong a need to confess. She probably thought it was a phase that would pass in time.

My next encounter with OCD happened when I was about thirteen. Where my OCD was between ages seven and thirteen is not clear. Maybe it was there in a mild form that was difficult to recognize or maybe it went into hibernation. It's common for OCD to this, especially in kids. The authors of several OCD memoirs describe similar experiences to mine where their OCD waxed and waned during their childhoods. They remember having specific symptoms for a while followed by a period, up to several years, where their lives returned to normal. Why this happens isn't clear, but I suspect that environmental stresses, such as those that routinely occur at school, in the home, or between peers, are involved. In other words, if life is going well, then maybe OCD can't find a stronghold to latch onto and as a result, fades away.

My (and Ray's) experience of childhood OCD is common, but not all who have OCD experience it at young ages. Some don't see an OCD symptom until adolescence or even early adulthood. Why we experience OCD at different times in our lives isn't clear but probably results from the differing ways in which OCD is caused. Some who have OCD, for example, may have inherited genes that cause them to experience OCD symptoms at a young age while others have OCD genes that are expressed only after puberty. Adding to this complexity is the endless variations of environments we live in. If a child who possesses the genetic predisposition for OCD is exposed, say, to a stressful environment, then their chances of developing this disorder at a young age is increased. If, however, the same child is allowed to live in a more stress-free environment, then it's likely that their OCD would take longer to spark.

OCD returned during my seventh grade year when I was experiencing stress in school. Specifically, I was having trouble understanding my science class. All the students were. The teacher had introduced a new way of teaching science and wasn't doing it well. For my fellow students, this was only an annoyance, but for me it was torture. The previous year I had discovered how to study and get straight A's. I liked that feeling, the one you get when the adults in your life praise you and tell you how good you are. But with this new class, I couldn't figure out how to do well and because of that, my worries started up again. I worried endlessly about the class, about how to get an A, and how disappointed I thought my parents would be if I failed to do well. To make matters worse, the teacher had implemented a new grading machine for our tests. When we finished with our test, we took it to our teacher, and he ran it through a machine that was located in the front of the classroom. Any wrong answer was "heard" by a strike like an old-fashioned typewriter key hitting the paper. For some kids, it was like listening to a machine gun when their paper went through. We could all guess each other's grade simply by listening when a test paper was sent through the machine. Many of my fellow students thought this was fun and teased each other, but to me, it was like a public shaming.

For that entire school year, I obsessed over my performance in my science class. My worry was constant, and it took over all aspects of my life. I tried to explain these concerns to my parents, but they couldn't understand why someone would obsess over a class to such an extent. They tried telling me that it wasn't worth worrying about, that my life wouldn't be decided by what happened during the seventh grade, and that they would always love me even if I failed all my classes. In other words, they tried desperately to reassure me. But with OCD, reassurance does nothing to help but instead, often spurs the OCD onto greater levels. I don't remember specifically how this OCD episode ended, but I suspect that it left me when the class was over, and I no longer had to worry about my grade. It's funny, but I can't even remember what grade I actually got in the class. I remember the worrying, but not the outcome of all that worrying.

After middle school, my OCD took on a more chronic, low-grade form. Instead of having specific, time-limited episodes, my OCD set in to stay, becoming such a part of me that I no longer realized that my thinking wasn't normal. Even though I realized that others went through life without as much anguish, it never occurred to me that my thinking could be changed. Instead, I faced each day, never at peace, and never feeling relaxed, happy, or confident. My worries were many and took on several forms. One of the main ones, however, was that I often endlessly replayed conversations in my mind looking for clues that I had offended someone or for something that I said that would make others not like me. Because of these worries, I would either avoid engaging in conversations or would shamelessly seek reassurance from others by saying such inane things as, "I hope I didn't offend you by what I just said; Did I just say something wrong?" I would also often quickly retreat when it was obvious that someone disagreed with me (ie, desperately trying to avoid any conflict). Needless to say, these behaviors cost me. Who would want to befriend or spend time with someone as quiet, shy, needy, and spineless as me? Ironically, OCD made me into someone others didn't want to spend time with, the very outcome I was compulsively trying to avoid.

For many years, I kept hoping that with age and experience my worries would disappear. All throughout college, medical school, pediatric residency, and finally, pediatric practice, I kept hoping that my thinking would normalize and that the confidence I saw in others would be mine. It never happened. Each day of my professional life was fraught with fears, specifically the fear that I would make a mistake that caused harm. As a pediatrician in a small community, there was never a lack of ideas for my OCD. My obsessions were many: Did I tell the parents everything that was important to keep their kids healthy? Did I make the right diagnosis, or did I make some horrible mistake that would cause a child's death or result in their disability? Did my patients and their parents even like me? In vain attempts to quell my ever-present anxieties, I compulsively trolled my textbooks or the internet looking for information, trying to reassure myself that I hadn't forgotten something, that I had made the right diagnosis and had recommended the right treatment. And, I was trying desperately not to let any of these insecurities show. After all, who wants to entrust their child's well being to someone as unsure as I felt? It was also important that I keep these OCD-ridden thoughts hidden from my fellow physicians and the nurses I worked with. How successful I was in this endeavor isn't clear, but I'm sure they saw it in me. As hard as I tried, there were times when my hesitations to take on extra work, my repeated questionings about certain patients, or my tendency to refer patients to specialists mostly likely raised suspicions about my ability to function.

How someone whose OCD centered on harm and its prevention survived a job where important decisions about children's health were made multiple times each day is an enigma. But somehow, I did it. It wasn't easy and many times, I wanted to quit. There were also times, about twice a year, when I did quit for several days, calling in sick and feigning a physical illness to cover the damage OCD was causing me. Whether my colleagues saw through these thinly-veiled attempts to hide my OCD they never let on; maybe they were too busy with their own lives to give me much thought or if they did, they dismissed my absences as a weakness.

Knowing that I obsessively worry about causing others harm, it would have made more sense for someone like me to choose a different job, one where the pace and intensity was such that I could take breaks where I needed or where my direct contact with others and their well being was not as frequent or intense. My life would have been easier, but I'm not convinced it would have been as complete. How I came to possess the fortitude to override my many misgivings about my abilities and forge ahead with such a difficult job will never be clear to me. Maybe I was lucky in that my brain had enough healthy pathways that could be used to overcome the OCD ones, or maybe I was just plain stubborn. Perhaps there was also a part of me that thought if I just kept facing down what scared me that eventually, it would all get better.

Adding to the myriad of difficulties my obsessions caused was yet another problem: People sometimes took advantage of my symptoms, specifically my compulsions to keep everyone happy with me. They didn't do this blatantly as in, "She's so anxious about being liked by everyone so maybe I could have her do whatever I want; She would never stand up for herself because she's so desperate to keep everyone happy so maybe I will have her do all the undesirable jobs." Instead, my vulnerabilities would become too much of a temptation for some, and they would use me for their own benefit. In a way, I don't blame them; it's useful having someone like me around. I was the kind of person, for example, who would take the blame if someone else accidently stepped on my foot. I would immediately apologize for my foot being in the wrong place where it was sure to be stepped on and even for yelping because of the pain. Whoever had made the mistake of stepping on my foot didn't have to feel any embarrassment or need to apologize. The end result was that I would limp away with a sore foot, feeling bad that I had caused a problem and obsess over how I had failed to prevent something bad from happening. Because of my tendencies, I became the depository for the bad feelings that others had. Some people around me even learned that all they had to do was to demonstrate their unhappiness, sometimes by only a frown or by giving me the silent treatment, and I would immediately change my behavior to better suit their desires. It was like I had no roots and was destined to blow wherever the wind (ie, the desires of others) took me.

I quit practicing medicine when Ray's OCD sparked to life and threatened to take over. Even though my own OCD had yet to be identified, I recognized his symptoms and knew that he was in trouble. If there was ever a time that he needed me to pay attention and not be wrapped up in my own world, this was it. Maybe others, especially those who don't have OCD or other mental conditions, could have taken care of their child's mental disorder and kept working as a physician, but not me. My handicaps were too big, and my fear of failure was too great. In a strange twist of fate, it was probably my own OCD that made me quit my practice. As Ray's OCD deepened, I obsessed about how to help him, how it was my responsibility to get him through, and how I couldn't face it if my son didn't get better and have a good life.

It took years of wrestling with my son's OCD before I realized my own problems with obsessions. Gradually, I learned to dissect my own thinking, unraveling those thoughts which were OCD-related and push them away. But, it took me a long time to reverse my decades-old habit and even today, I sometimes fall back into my old thinking. My OCD pathways remain with me and on occasion, they fire up, testing whether or not they can gather some momentum and cause trouble. It usually doesn't take me long, however, to detect OCD's hand in my thinking and correct my course.

An example of the presence of my lingering OCD pathways occurred recently when my family and I were traveling on a cruise ship. I was standing near a hot tub when I suddenly heard a woman's voice crying out that something was wrong with her husband and that she needed help. The physician in me responded, assessed the situation, and quickly concluded that the poor man had simply passed out. By the time I had reached his side, he was regaining his senses and trying to reassure his distraught wife. We talked for a while; he quickly recovered; and they returned to their cabin as if nothing unusual had happened. After seeing them off, I also went on my way. But within about an hour, my mind started turning over thoughts like, "Did you really think through what happened, maybe he's really sick, and you missed it; maybe he will die, and it'll be your fault." After about three rounds of this thinking and feeling an ominous dread welling up in me, I understood what was happening. My OCD had been engaged and was trying to gain some traction. So instead of accommodating it, I turned to it, personally addressing it and said, "Maybe you are right. Maybe that man will die tonight even though I seriously doubt it. I'm a competent physician, and I know how to recognize a simple fainting spell. But even if he does die, it's not my fault." With these simple thoughts, my OCD retreated and didn't attempt to return. (By the way, I saw the man the next day, and he looked as healthy as ever.)

My OCD was eventually tamed using the skills we learned during the treatment of Ray's OCD. As we figured out how to deal with Ray's OCD, I realized that the same ideas would also help me change my thinking. But, it wasn't enough. It's one thing to know what to do and an entirely different one to muster the strength and persistence to do it. After Ray's OCD had been beaten back and we were focusing on how to rebuild his life, I decided to see a psychiatrist for help. Ray still needed me to help him figure out his next steps, but I was spent. My mental energy had been drained away in the fight to help him, and I couldn't find any way to regain my strength. I needed help, so I dragged my sorry self into a psychiatrist's office. In a way, I did this more for Ray than for me; I was still worrying about how it was my responsibility to help him and that any failure would entirely be my fault.

The psychiatrist diagnosed me with dysthymia (a low-grade, chronic depression) and gave me an antidepressant (Zoloft). I took it, gradually felt lighter, and dug in again to help Ray. Buoyed by this newly-found sustenance, life moved along easier, and Ray once again had his loyal companion to help him figure out his next steps. And, I also had the mental reserve to finally beat back my own OCD. Even though my psychiatrist didn't tag OCD as my current problem, we both acknowledged the role it had in creating my depression. I had become so beaten down by OCD that I now acted more like someone with depression than someone who has OCD. With the help of medication, I could identify what damage OCD had done to my life, what patterns of thinking were OCD related, and what interventions I needed to use to correct my aberrant brain pathways. In other words, instead of only surviving life, I could now live it. It was like I had finally found a way to pull myself into a lifeboat instead of always hanging onto the side, hoping that someday I would be allowed a seat where I would feel safe.

Ray doesn't remember any effects that my OCD might have caused him when he was growing up. This isn't surprising; children often can't see their parent's struggles. They are too busy figuring out their own lives.

ΔΔΔΔ

It is hard to say whether or not my mom having OCD seriously affected me while growing up. In fact, I do not remember any single case where I noticed her having OCD. However, it is possible that because my mom had OCD, she was less inclined to spend time with me when I was younger and give me the support I may have needed.

Like I mentioned, I have no memory of seeing my mom undergo any symptoms of OCD. I never saw her frequently wash her hands or double check things, but I did sense that she worried a lot. Every time she came home from her work as a doctor, she would be completely exhausted and sometimes, was tentative to spend time with me. Understandably, being a doctor is hard work, but I sensed that it overwhelmed her at times. This excessive worry was probably due to the strains OCD put on her because it made her worry obsessively and uncontrollably about things. However, it is hard for me to say how much my mom's OCD had to do with how I was raised or how my OCD developed.

However, my mom having OCD provided some advantages for me. When I first started having signs of OCD, like asking for reassurances that I was not going to die, my mom recognized the thoughts I had as thoughts she had also experienced. Even though she did not know what to do about them at the time, she knew that something was wrong. Then, when my OCD got worse when I was a teenager, she recognized it as something that had to be dealt with and decided to quit her job to help me. I have heard stories of people who go years dealing with OCD without truly knowing what they are facing. Without a doubt, one of the most important steps to dealing with OCD is recognizing your thoughts as a product of OCD. Once you can do this, then you can really start fighting back your OCD.

Ray's OCD Story

In our family, OCD was first identified by name because of my son, Ray. In him, it no longer remained hidden but showed itself in all its ugliness, vileness, and unmercifulness. Whereas both my mother and I stumbled along in life, not knowing the name of what held us back or even that we had an identifiable condition, the situation was different for Ray. His symptoms were stronger, more pronounced, and they affected his life in more obvious ways.

Ray was about fourteen when his OCD dug in and threatened to take over his life in an ominous way. It was during the summer break between his eight grade and freshmen year of high school when his OCD flared and refused to let up. We knew what we were dealing with during this time because OCD had tried on several previous occasions to take root and grow into something more substantial. But for reasons that are still not really understood, OCD didn't find any real ground during those previous episodes and had withered away.

The first time I remember OCD-like symptoms in Ray occurred when he was about five. During a period of about two weeks, I noticed that he would run into the bathroom and wash his hands several times in an hour. This didn't happen every day; on some days, he didn't wash his hands at all, but on others, it was a constant activity for him. When asked, he couldn't say why he was doing this, and just when I was starting to wonder what his behaviors meant, he stopped. All during this time, he didn't look anxious, and he didn't say that he was afraid of germs or that he would get sick if he didn't wash his hands. He looked happy and in between his hand washings, he was as active, engaged, and playful as before. Was this the first spark of his OCD or was it just a normal fascination with running water that a little kid was experiencing? How many other kids do something similar but don't go on to have OCD? We will never know if this short-lived, hand washing episode was caused by some nascent OCD circuits trying to fire. And, even if we had recognized the behavior as OCD, would there have been anything to do about it?

For three years between the ages of five and eight, Ray didn't experience anything that could be remotely identified as OCD. He went to school, played with his friends, and did all the things most kids do at that age. But around eight, he started asking me strange questions like, "I just touched this wall with my hand, do you think that everything will be all right?" He was also very concerned that he and the people around him might die and asked constantly for reassurance that it wouldn't happen. Ray also remembers being very worried that something had fallen off his bed and that he would check several times before he could relax enough to fall asleep. I didn't know what to make of his worries and did what most parents would do in such a situation: I tried to alleviate his fears by reassuring him that everything was all right. But as anyone who has ever dealt with OCD knows, providing reassurance does nothing and in fact, often worsens someone's symptoms. And, that's exactly what happened to us. The more reassurance I gave Ray, the more he requested it. I was unknowingly feeding the OCD monster when my intentions had been simply to quell my son's anxieties. Ray gradually moved from accepting my reassurance to requesting that I guarantee him that nothing bad would happen. In time, he then moved to requesting a super guarantee and when that wasn't enough, a super-super guarantee. Finally, by the end, he was demanding that I give him a super-super-super guarantee.

Ray's anxiety at age eight was the first time I recognized that his behaviors were more than just a normal phase, but I didn't identify his symptoms as OCD. Like most parents, I wasn't sure what to do but hoped that it would go away with time. It did. Within a couple of months, Ray's anxieties about death and his need for constant reassurance faded, and he resumed his life like nothing had happened.   Life forged on, and we all soon forgot this episode. I have often wondered if it would have made any difference to Ray if this episode had been identified for what it was: An OCD flare. Maybe if I had been more aware of this, then Ray's future OCD episodes could have been more quickly identified and treated. Maybe the suffering he was to undergo as a teenager could have been lessened if I had thought harder about what he had experienced when he was eight. We will never know for sure, but I have often felt tremendous guilt for not understanding more about OCD when Ray was younger.

As expected, Ray doesn't remember as much as I do from this time, but he does remember some of what he experienced.

ΔΔΔΔ

The first time I remember having any signs of OCD occurred when I was about eight years old. It was shortly after a trip to Hong Kong to visit my grandmother when I started having strange thoughts about death. I would worry that any small action on my part could elicit some supernatural cause of death to my family or me. For example, I remember once touching my feet to a wall while watching television and immediately, I was bombarded with obsessions about my whole family dying. I had to go to my mom immediately and beg for a guarantee that we would all be okay. My mom, not recognizing that my worries were resulting from OCD, reassured me that nothing would go wrong. After each time I got a reassurance, however, I became more and more skeptical about whether or not my mom really knew if everything was going to be all right. Because of this, I began asking for super guarantees, followed by super-super guarantees, and so forth.

During this time, I also spent at least half an hour each night checking around my room to make sure that things were in order. Every night I slept with around twenty stuffed animals, and I would be plagued with thoughts suggesting that some of my stuffed animals had fallen off my bed and onto the floor. I would worry that these stuffed animals would be scared, and I would vividly imagine what it would be like if I were in the stuffed animal's place. So, I would do a quick check around my bed and lay back down. Sure enough though, like an annoying fly, the thought would come back, and there I was checking again.

It was also around this time that my mom realized something was wrong and that these thoughts were not normal. I, too, had sensed that something was not quite right but being eight, didn't worry too much about it. In fact, I don't really remember being too affected by this early OCD episode.

ΔΔΔΔ

After the episode when he was eight, Ray's OCD quieted down and didn't show up again until he was about eleven. Where it was hiding during those three years between episodes isn't clear, but for that time period, Ray didn't have any identifiable symptoms. When he was about to turn eleven, however, OCD made itself known again and this time, it was larger, more intense, and unmistakably a problem. This was the episode that made me pay attention, realize that my son was in trouble, and forced us to admit that something was terribly wrong. There was no waiting this episode out; it was time to act. The problem was I didn't know what to do.

Ray's OCD roared back to life during a period when our family was undergoing stress, not the bad kind of stress, such as impending divorces, financial problems, or job losses, but the more benign kind. We had been living in Shanghai, China for about a year and were preparing to return home. My husband, who is Chinese, had wanted us to live in China for a while so that Ray could spend time with his grandmother. During our time in China, Ray had attended a Chinese school; I practiced pediatrics in a Chinese hospital; and my husband taught in a university. Ray did well, despite his challenges on not initially understanding the language that was spoken at school and at being teased because he was not Chinese. He was never outright bullied, but he did have to deal with looking and sounding different from his peers. He bravely faced each day, rarely showed any anxiety, and remained active. The only concern he mentioned was that he wondered if his friends back in the U.S. would forget him and would they still be his friends when he got home.

About a month before we returned home, Ray mentioned that he was having some strange thoughts that bothered him a lot. I don't remember exactly when he first told me about his "bad thoughts." I was too busy with my work and with preparing to move back home to really hear what he was telling me. And, I was probably hoping that this episode of strange thoughts would go away like they had before. They didn't, buy instead grew larger and more ominous every day. Within a short time, Ray's symptoms became large enough to demand my attention. I couldn't ignore them any longer for they were now a constant presence in our home and were loud enough to drown out all other sounds. It had finally dawned on me that it was time to address the proverbial elephant in the room, who had somehow marched into our home, plopped himself down, and refused to budge. And, when I finally looked that elephant in the eye, asked him what he was doing here, and what it would take to convince him to leave, he simply laughed in my face. He knew we were no match for him.

Even though I had listened to Ray endlessly confess this thoughts, I only had a vague notion of what they consisted of. Ray had fallen into a habit where he would tell me that he was having a thought and then wait for me to reassure him that he was still a good person. I was still so naïve to OCD and how it functions that I readily gave him that reassurance simply because he had asked for it and because the relief he felt after receiving it was obvious. It was like he was telling me that he was in physical pain and was asking for morphine. Why wouldn't I give it to him? I was his mother and wasn't it my responsibility to alleviate his pain in any way possible? It made sense to me at that time that I should give him the reassurance he asked for, whenever he asked for it. It didn't occur to me that I needed to look closer at the source of his pain instead of just "medicating" it.

Ray's obsessions during this episode were sexual in nature. What exactly they were, Ray either wouldn't or couldn't tell me. Even trying to explain his obsessions would trigger them, which was something he definitely wanted to avoid. With time and persistent digging, however, I realized that his "thoughts" were multidimensional in nature. Sometimes they consisted of actual thoughts like, "I want to have sex with that woman I just saw in the street; I wonder what that woman sitting next to me would look like without her clothes." On other times, it was more like a feeling or sensation he had. He could never say for sure what these feelings were really like, but I often wondered if they consisted of sexual urges, such as a tingling or other sensation in the genital area. Even though such sensations are universal in that everyone experiences them (often multiple times) on a daily basis, Ray's OCD had convinced him that such feelings meant that he was a bad person. A third element to Ray's bad thoughts consisted of images that sometimes flashed through his mind. Here again, he could never say exactly what those pictures looked like, but it's likely they consisted of sexual matters, such as images of sexual acts and naked bodies. Ray never said which of the three ways (ie, thoughts, sensations, or images) were most prominent in his OCD; it's probable that all three were involved interchangeably.

Ray remembers some of this time, but not to the same extent that I do. I have never found this lack of remembrance surprising, and I even think it's somewhat protective. Maybe our brains selectively edit out those times when we have pain, especially childhood pain. He does, however, remember one incident which happened early on during this OCD episode.

ΔΔΔΔ

While I was living with my parents in China for a year, we took a trip with some family friends to a neighboring village near Shanghai. During the whole trip, I could not keep my mind off of one simple comment I had made to my friend. We were talking about funny names, and I brought up my old kindergarten teacher whose name was Mrs. Ball (a name that can easily be made into a dirty joke). To an eleven year old, these jokes are hilarious, and I found it incredibly funny at the time, too. However, soon after I made that joke, creeping thoughts bothered me daily about how inappropriate and disgusting such a joke was. I could not enjoy a single moment of my life because of how much I was plagued at the idea that I was a horrible kid for making such a joke. One day while we were standing in line at a McDonald's, I had finally had enough, and I confessed to my mom about my joke. She, of course, dismissed it and told me that there was nothing to worry about.

ΔΔΔΔ

By the time we finally reached home, Ray's OCD was gaining momentum like a runaway train. Several times each hour he would search for me so that he could confess yet another "bad thought," and on several occasions, he would curl into a fetal position and cry like his heart was breaking. Many times, he asked why this was happening to him and what had he done to deserve such

42

pain. Not yet understanding how to handle OCD, we tried several interventions, hoping that one would finally break through his pain and ease it. On the weekends, we went out and did things together, like watching a movie, talking a walk, or eating out. We did these activities hoping that the distractions they provided would magically replace the uncomfortable thoughts that were dominating Ray's mind. On the occasional day that I had free, we would stay home, laze about, taking naps or watching TV; maybe if all stress and expectations were removed from Ray's environment, then he could use all his energy to fight back and deal with his anxieties. When these simple ideas failed, I knew it was time to try something more radical.

Ever since Ray was born I had worked long hours because in medicine, that's what required of you. But, when I saw how miserable Ray was and how nothing we were trying was helping, I realized that my hospital could always find another pediatrician but how was Ray to find another mother who would dig deep and help him through his troubles? For the first time in Ray's life, I chose him over my work. I quit being a pediatrician and turned my attention to Ray. Weathering all the upheavals this decision spurred wasn't easy; I had agreed to come back so the parents of my patients were upset; my family had yet to understand what was happening to Ray so they were mystified that I was giving up a career that took years to attain; and I was lost. For many of us, our careers define us, telling the world who we are and what we have to offer. In the very least, our jobs give us a place to be each day and a host of people to interact with. But, now I was giving all that up in an attempt to help Ray with his troubles.

Even before we could both adjust to our new arrangement (ie, me being home all the time), Ray's OCD plunged ahead and took on more bizarre forms. In addition to yelling out "bad thought" and demanding that I give him reassurance, his OCD actually started to string ideas together, not exactly into a story, but close. One day, for example, Ray looked at me and asked, "How do you know with absolute certainty that I didn't drug you into unconsciousness and then sexually molest you?" At another time, he wondered, "How do you know for sure that I haven't molested someone who had walked out of a nearby cornfield and then disappeared back into it before you noticed their presence?" It was like he was no longer sure about what was real; his sense of reality had become blurred. Before he made these types of statements, I had been merely worried, but now I was terrified. What was happening to his mind? Was he slipping into some kind of psychosis where it would be harder to reach him?

Maybe I should have hauled Ray into the nearest emergency room after hearing him say such strange and unhinged things, but I didn't. Maybe I should have treated him like the emergency he was rapidly becoming, but even as scared as I was with Ray's symptoms, I also feared what our local mental health professionals might do. For years, I had tried to get good psychiatric care for my pediatric patients but had felt that on many occasions, they were let down. Their parents often returned from those visits with diagnoses they couldn't understand, multiple medications that made their kids zombie-like, and many times, they refused to go back for a follow-up visit. I also worried about the possibility that a psychiatrist would insist that Ray be admitted to a local inpatient facility, a step which I felt would be useless and possibly, even harmful to him. In short, I had no faith in our local mental health community. They had lost it years ago, and there was no way that I was putting Ray in their care.

As I was trying to find a viable plan to get Ray help, something unbelievable happened: Ray slowly improved. Instead of his symptoms careening towards a cliff, they slowed down, lost their momentum, and even started to fade a little. Why this happened wasn't clear, but I was grateful for the breathing room. We will never know, but I think the slowdown occurred because we had eliminated as much stress from our home as we could and had established some new routines. I had stopped trying to reestablish myself at a job and had stopped pushing Ray to do things that he didn't want to do. Because he had spent the previous year in China, I was worried that he was behind in certain subjects at school and had been pushing him to study. Of course, these attempts were going badly. Who could possibly study math, social studies, or science when their mind is swirling with obsessions? Once we stopped trying so hard to get things done, Ray found a new reserve of mental energy that he could now use to deal with his obsessions. And as time went on that summer, he slowly pushed back his symptoms so that when fall arrived, he was ready for school.

Adding to our massive confusion during this time was the problem that we didn't have a name to what was afflicting Ray. Even though I was a pediatrician and had some training in psychiatry, I still didn't recognize that what was happening to Ray was called OCD. I just thought he was overly anxious and maybe a diagnosis, like general anxiety disorder, was appropriate for him. Like most physicians, my exposure to OCD had been limited to a few sentences in a textbook or to a few minutes in some long-ago lecture. And, what I remembered was some vague idea of people who couldn't stop washing their hands or were stuck on certain numbers. Nowhere in any of my books was there information telling me that OCD can take on many, different forms including the sexual one that had overtaken Ray's mind. The other problem was that I assumed that in OCD, the compulsions would be obvious like hand washing or counting. Ray didn't do anything like this. The proverbial light bulb went on a few months later when I was reading a review article on anxiety disorders in pediatrics. There it was in black and write: OCD can take on many forms including sexuality. And, compulsions can consist of things like repeatedly confessing or incessantly asking for reassurance. I had no doubt after reading that article that Ray had OCD. At least now, we had a name and a more definite direction to look for information.

Learning about OCD after Ray's had cooled down was a little like closing the barn door after the horse had already run away, but I figured it was still a good idea to keep thinking about it. Somehow, I knew that OCD wasn't gone for good and that we had better prepare ourselves for the fight that was sure to come. Like the adage says: Know thy enemy. OCD was our enemy, and if we were ever to have a decent chance in dealing with it, we needed to learn everything we could. This idea, of course, is easier to think about than to actually execute. How much knowledge is enough? How many books does one have to read before becoming an expert? In my naivety, I made one of my many mistakes: I actually thought that after reading only two books on OCD that I understood it and was prepared to handle it when it showed up again. After all, the books had been written by experts in the field and surely they had packed all the essential information in their books that parents would need. I thought that by following through with the suggestions in these books that we could successfully handle any flare ups of Ray's OCD. In retrospect, I realize that this idea was like preparing to go to war by gathering up several pitchforks and placing them by the door. Their presence would make me feel more secure, but for actual fighting, they would be useless.

Our failure to adequately prepare for OCD's return was also fueled by a simple observation: Ray's OCD had backed down without us doing anything other than decreasing the stress in his life. Even though Ray's OCD had become severe and had markedly affected his life, it had died down almost as fast as it had flared. Maybe all we had to do for any future return of his OCD was to simply wait it out. Maybe for Ray, his OCD would always burn itself out if given enough time. Admittedly, I liked this idea. It was comforting to think that OCD would just go away and leave us alone after a while. Needless to say, this thinking was wrong, naive, and even dangerous.

Throughout the next three years, Ray's OCD didn't regain the strength it previously had, but it didn't disappear either. He still had symptoms, but they were mild. Every so often, he would tell me he was having an obsession, but he never appeared particularly worried about it. He would also have flares of OCD around times of transitions, like going from to school to summer break or when under stress. But, his OCD would always cool back down once the stress or transition had passed. If Ray's OCD had remained in this form, (ie, relatively quiet and easily handled), we would have considered ourselves extremely lucky. We had already seen what OCD could do and didn't want to ever deal with it again.

Ray's OCD storm started up again during the summer before he was to start high school. Since he often had minor OCD flares with the beginning of breaks, I wasn't too worried and hoped that as the summer wore on, his symptoms would return to their usual low levels. But, they didn't. Day by day, he got worse. Instead of telling me that he was having a bad thought several times per day, he had progressed to telling me several times per hour. And, the way he was now telling me had changed. Instead of just saying it almost like an afterthought, he was now practically yelling it. He also made sure that I responded to him where before, just saying it out loud was enough. He needed to hear me say that it was all right for him to have such thoughts and that he was still a good person, even though his thoughts made him feel otherwise. During this episode, however, my reassurances gradually lost their power, and to help him deal with his awful feelings, Ray added another compulsion: Hand washing. Ray's hand washing wasn't because he feared germs and the sicknesses they convey, but because he felt guilty about his obsessions and somehow, the washing gave him relief from that guilt.

Throughout that summer, Ray's OCD marched steadily ahead, and nothing we did could stop it. I kept hoping that it would relent in its intensity but instead, it kept growing larger. His symptoms multiplied, gradually encompassing every aspect of our lives. At one point, it seemed like a new obsession or compulsion appeared almost hourly. He went from washing his hands out of guilt to washing them because he thought he was spreading sexual material throughout his environment, and it was paramount to him that he not be responsible for this. His obsessions, for reasons we have never figured out, continued their focus on sexuality, much like they did when he was eleven. But contrary to when he was younger, they were more numerous, varied in their presentation, and unlimited in their ability to divide and morph into yet another form. By the time we cried uncle at the end of the year, Ray's OCD was in complete control of his life.

All aspects of sexuality triggered Ray's obsessions, both external clues and internal bodily sensations. Every female he encountered, including those in movies or on television programs, would cause a wave of obsessions and compulsions. At his worst, he couldn't bear to look at a woman or girl in any context without experiencing what looked like shocks of pure pain. He also went to extremes to avoid any of these ubiquitous triggers, a situation which is impossible to attain unless one completely retreats from the world. He would, for example, move as far away as possible from a woman if he thought that he was about to meet her in a store aisle or in a hallway. He would move as close as he could to the opposite wall and slink along there until he felt better. I often thought that he looked like a trapped animal, desperately trying to escape. And, if a situation arose where it was impossible for him to escape being in the proximity of a woman, he would start obsessing that he had somehow, unknowingly, and purposely bumped into her in a sexual manner. Many times when I was with Ray in a store or walking with him on the street, he would suddenly insist that we leave because he couldn't deal with all the triggers that were bombarding him.

Even though Ray's OCD focused mainly on females, it eventually grew to include other aspects of sexuality. Not surprisingly, he would occasionally say that his obsessions included males. He never said for certain what this meant, but I assumed that his OCD was causing him to have similar thoughts about men as it did about women (eg, sexual acts, exposed bodies, and physical sensations). But, these types of thoughts never reached the same intensity of those that concerned females. More unusual, however, was his obsessions that concerned our household cats. On occasion, he would blurt out that he had just looked at one of the cat's anal areas and that it was causing him extreme anxiety. I imagine that if we had had other household pets, such as dogs, rabbits, or mice, Ray's OCD would have eventually involved those species as well. Of all his sexual obsessions, though, the ones that caused him the hardest time were the ones concerning children, mainly those who were younger than him at the time. When his obsessions combined children with sexuality, it became even more painful for him to bear. Previous to having these obsessions, Ray had already felt like he was some sort of sexual pervert, but now that his obsessions involved children, he worried incessantly that he was a pedophile who shouldn't be allowed to live.

Ray's OCD also invaded our home so that it no longer provided him with any sense of comfort or reprieve. At one point, he considered every inch of our floors, every doorknob, every piece of furniture and countertop as contaminated. His contamination fears, however, had nothing to do with germs but with sexual material, which consisted mainly of semen but also of any type of secretion that had been emitted from his genital area. Strangely, one of the main sources of the feared sexual material was located in one particular bathroom that was situated close to our kitchen area and was the one that was often used by guests. Even though this bathroom was regularly cleaned, Ray's OCD had convinced him that sexual material, namely semen, remained in the bathroom from a time when he was younger and had freely experimented with his body (ie, masturbated). In his OCD-twisted mind, the semen that remained within that bathroom was spread throughout the house by anyone who dared use the bathroom. If, for example, Ray observed someone coming out of the bathroom and then sitting on a couch, he would refuse to sit on that couch. Or, if he thought someone had walked on a certain area of the floor after using the bathroom, he would then try to avoid the same area. His focus on this particular bathroom had become so intense and encompassing that we dubbed it, "the evil bathroom."

Eventually, Ray didn't even have to directly observe anyone having contact with the "evil bathroom," just the slightest hint of possible contamination was enough for him to deem yet another area, surface, or object as "dirty." Even several degrees of removal from that bathroom were still strong enough to trigger his anxiety (eg, a book bag might be targeted as contaminated because it was sitting on the floor and might have been walked on by one the cats who might have been petted by someone who might have used the "evil bathroom" and touched some surface that might have been in contact with something as bad as semen). With this convoluted thinking, it didn't take Ray's OCD long before it convinced him that his entire home and everyone in it (or had ever been in it) wasn't safe. The only room where his OCD wasn't as forbidding was his own bedroom, but even there, it maintained a definite and looming presence.

Ray's Compulsions

Desperately trying to find some relief Ray did what most people who have OCD do: He turned towards compulsions. Similar to his early OCD episodes, he would endlessly ask me for reassurance that he wasn't a bad person for having his thoughts or that he wouldn't do something that might cause harm to someone else. He also resumed his compulsion of yelling out "bad thought," several times each hour, which was his shorthand version of reassurance seeking. Even though I could sometimes get away from overtly responding to these endless outbursts, he would make sure that I had heard. And, when he wasn't absolutely certain that I had heard his words, he would simply repeat them or get my attention if he suspected that I wasn't listening. Many times, for example, Ray would elbow me during a movie, lean as close to my ear as possible, and whisper "bad thought." In these cases, if I didn't respond by either moving away from him or by shaking my head, he would repeat himself until he was sure I had heard.

Like his obsessions, Ray's compulsions during this time were more intense and varied. In addition to his constant reassurance seeking, he added other compulsions, sometimes in succession to each other and on some occasions, they were added simultaneously. Most of these new compulsions, however, were centered on one main idea: Washing. Ray started by washing his hands, a compulsion that is shared by many who have OCD (one estimate is that 50% of those who have OCD will have hand washing as a compulsion). And like his fellow sufferers of OCD, his hand washing didn't just stay in one form but morphed, almost daily, in intensity, frequency, and in procedure. At his worst, Ray would wash his hands several times per hour. He would also count the squirts of hand soap until he reached the number that gave him a sense of security, a number that skyrocketed to absurdity within a short time. At one point, Ray was using so much soap at school that a janitor had posted a sign in the boy's bathroom stating that since the soap was vanishing too quickly, he wasn't going to replace it for a while and for whoever was causing this soap disappearance to please stop. At home, of course, the situation wasn't any better. In my ignorance and in an attempt to keep Ray from melting down, I supplied his required soap in several bathrooms and by the kitchen sink. The amount he used was unimaginable; it would have been easier just to have bought a truckload of the stuff, unloaded it into our home, and mainlined it into each faucet.

Within a short time of starting his hand washing, Ray bore one of the most obvious physical signs of OCD: Red, chapped hands. No amount of lotion, cream, or gel can ever improve this condition, mainly because it never stays on long enough to help. Several times I wondered what his teachers, friends, or even our family thought when they saw those lobster hands of his. Did they think he had a skin condition and that he needed to see a dermatologist? Maybe they assumed that since it was so obvious that I was taking care of it and felt no need to ask him what was going on. And since Ray kept his other symptoms well hidden, it probably never occurred to anyone that he had a condition like OCD. Also, it's likely that even if someone, who had experience with OCD, did catch on and ask him about it, he probably would have denied having his obsessions and made up some plausible reason for his hands looking so bad.

Ray quickly became tolerant to what relief his hand washing provided and started washing more of his body in a desperate attempt to keep feeling relaxed. He went from scrubbing his hands to washing his wrists, forearms, and eventually, his arms. When this level of washing inevitably failed to suffice, he threw handfuls of water on both of his ankles and feet each time he did his washing ritual. By the end of most evenings, water would stream off the kitchen rugs when they were picked up; it was like they had been dunked in water and then returned to the floor. The only exposed part of his body he wasn't washing during these rituals was his face, head, and neck.

Because Ray's OCD centered on sexual matters and focused heavily on the presence of sexual material, it didn't take long for him to start showering several times per day. He obsessively worried that the secretions from his genital area was causing harm to others and that he needed to protect them by continually cleaning his body. During this time, it was common for Ray to take up to four showers a day with each one requiring a complete change of clothes. In the OCD world, this isn't too extreme. Some with OCD will take hours-long showers, multiple times a day. I read a story about one man with OCD who was kicked out of his apartment because he continually ran his shower, using so much water that it came to the attention of the building manager, who then insisted that the man leave because of his huge and unexplainable water usage.

With Ray taking so many showers each day, the pile of laundry became mountainous. He would sometimes also add to that pile by inexplicably deciding that he needed to change his clothes even if a shower hadn't been involved. There were even occasions when he would dump clean clothes into a hamper because he had had an obsession while his hand was on the clothes pile. Somehow, his OCD mind convinced him that all the clothes in that pile were now dirty just because he had an obsession while touching them. Yet another addition to the ever-present laundry pile was an almost daily presence of Ray's sheets and blankets. He had become so worried that bodily fluids had leaked out onto his bedding while he was asleep and that they would cause havoc on the world in unimaginable ways unless they were immediately washed away. I tried to circumvent some of the laundry by telling Ray that I would take care of it while he was at school but of course, that failed. His OCD had learned not to trust me. Ray had to be the one who put his bedding or his "dirty" clothes into the washing machine. He had to see it safely in the washer with the lid closed before he could move on. If, on the rare occasion, my hands did touch any of his laundry and he saw it happen, he would immediately insist that I wash my hands with a large amount of soap and then thoroughly dry them. When I think back at this time in Ray's OCD, it's hard to imagine that I had time for anything else other than doing his OCD's bidding.

Unfortunately, his body parts, clothes, and bedding were not the only things Ray insisted on washing. At least those things could stand soap and water and not break down or disintegrate. As his world gradually became more contaminated, Ray washed all sorts of items that were never meant to face water. His homework and band music, for example, were often subjected to "washings," and electronic items, such as cell phones, remote controls, calculators, and computer keyboards, were needlessly exposed to water. The paper items were routinely destroyed as most do when placed in water, and as for the electronic items, some made it through Ray's OCD but others were seriously damaged. Sometimes, Ray realized that a certain item might not do well if cleaned and if he was to have continued use of that item, he needed to be careful. On these occasions, Ray would perform a virtual, as opposed to an actual, cleaning by simply dabbing a moistened cloth on the item instead of using soap and water.

Lucky for us, most of Ray's "cleaning" involved our own things and only rarely, encroached on the property of others. This most likely resulted because Ray actively avoided touching items that belonged to others. He feared that he would feel responsible for any "contamination" of those items that his OCD insisted had occurred. One time, however, his system failed, and he ended up holding a friend's cell phone, which he then immediately felt had become "dirty." His friend had wanted Ray to use his cell phone to call another friend and had tossed his phone to Ray who instinctively caught it. Of course, Ray's

OCD immediately insisted that the phone required cleaning before being returned to its owner. To deal with this situation, Ray made some lame excuse, such as wanting to call from the bathroom and then dashed off to the nearest bathroom where he could find a way to decontaminate the phone. Fortunately, Ray found a way to do this which both satisfied his OCD and allowed the cell phone to remain functioning. Whenever I think about this incident, I'm relieved that Ray didn't solve his problem in a more dramatic fashion such as "accidently" dropping the phone in a toilet or sink full of water or somehow "losing" the phone in a garbage can. Like many with OCD, Ray could often leash his OCD when the consequences of listening to it were embarrassing or could cause him losses he didn't want to bear.

When asked about his compulsions, Ray remembers many of his reassurance-seeking ones and of course, the endless washing.

ΔΔΔΔ

The first compulsion I remember was repeatedly asking my mom whether or not something bad was going to happen. This happened when I was around eight years old, and it was the first time my OCD came about. Basically, I would ask for a guarantee that everything was going to be okay, shortly followed by a super guarantee and then a super-super-super guarantee. The amount of supers I would add only increased the more my mom reassured me.

Another compulsion I remember having was when we were living in China when I was around eleven years old. This compulsion was also one that I had when I was younger. Specifically, I was afraid that things might fall off my bed, such as pillows and beanie babies. At night, I would sleep with close to twenty stuffed animals on my bed, and I would worry that one of them would fall off and become "lonely." Therefore, before I went to bed each night, I would

55

check to make sure that nothing had fallen off my bed, and I would do this around ten to fifteen times. This compulsion was not severe, and my mom doesn't even remember it. However, I realize now that what I was doing during that time was probably related to OCD.

Later in China that year, I began having obsessions that were the first signs of my sexually-related OCD. It was during this time that I started confessing to my mom about my "bad thoughts." After we returned home, I continued having my sexual obsessions, and I relentlessly asked my mom for reassurance that I was a good person and not one who was amoral. I also incessantly confessed to her all the thoughts I was having and told her of all the possible ways that I might have hurt someone. I remember one time when I had visited my friend's home and had become obsessed with the possibility that I had done something sexual with his sister. Of course, I knew that I hadn't done anything bad, but my mind kept telling me I did. To deal with these thoughts, I painfully confessed to my mom and did so repeatedly.

The next step my compulsions took was washing. I first began washing my hands because of my sexual obsessions but then gradually, started washing other parts of my body, such as my arms and feet. I washed after having any sexual thought or when my OCD convinced me that I had somehow come into contact with sexual material, such as semen. During this time, I was also strangely obsessed over one particular bathroom in our home, and a lot of my washing resulted because of those obsessions.

There was a time when I had no OCD-related sexual thoughts and when I frequently masturbated in a specific bathroom. When my OCD became focused on sexuality, it targeted that bathroom because of my fear of "leftover" semen that could possibly be lurking somewhere in there. Eventually, my OCD convinced me that other people, who had gone into that bathroom, were spreading the semen around the house. Because of these obsessions, I *started washing my feet after stepping on places on the floor that I thought were contaminated with semen; I started opening doors with pieces of paper after my mom had opened that door (because I feared that she had used the bathroom I so feared); and I avoided any contact with my cats (since my mom had petted them).*

Avoidance of Triggers

During the time when Ray's OCD was active, he engaged in another technique that is commonly used by those whose OCD is raging. He actively avoided, or tried to, anything that might trigger his obsessions and hence, his unrestrained need to perform his compulsions. For Ray, this avoidance mainly consisted of trying not to have contact with any surface, object, or person that might trigger his bad thoughts or be contaminated with sexual material. At his worst, this list included just about everything and everyone in his world. Trying to exist in such a world is impossible, but Ray faced the challenges every day. It's hard for those who don't deal with OCD to imagine the difficulties one faces when trying to maneuver in a world that looks and feels so wrong and threatening. It also takes an amazing degree of creativity and imagination to find one's way through such a maze. I've often wondered how much progress could be made against OCD if those who have it were convinced to use their creativity as a force to face down their OCD instead of using it to help them avoid their triggers.

Ray often amazed me by how he avoided his triggers. Because his OCD didn't allow him to touch doorknobs, for example, he couldn't open a door when he needed to get through it. At school, when he needed to get into his classroom he would nonchalantly hang around the door, pretending he was doing something, such as tying his shoe or digging through his school bag, and wait until someone else opened the door. At home, where he felt more comfortable letting his OCD out, he would often rage at me until I gave up and opened a door for him. If I refused, he would either yell louder or would find a barrier, such as piece of paper or napkin, and use it to open the door. For the doors in public bathrooms, Ray would often kick the door open or wait until someone else opened it. Car doors were also a problem for Ray. If he possibly could, he would find ways to manipulate someone into opening the door for him. A favorite trick of his was to gather up everything he could in the car, such as his books, papers, coats, and then claim that his hands were too full to open the door. In these cases, it almost seemed rude not to open the door for him. After all, we routinely open doors for those whose hands are full. Ray knew this tendency and often used it to his OCD's advantage.

The floors in our home were another area where Ray's avoidance to his OCD triggers was obvious. Because he considered most areas on the floor as contaminated, he wasn't comfortable walking on them. To get from one place to another, he would jump on his tiptoes like he was being forced to walk on hot coals. How he decided where to jump I have never figured out. My best guess was that he was trying to minimize all floor contact by moving fast and by using only his tiptoes. He also never jumped in a straight line; maybe he thought that if he varied his direction, he would lessen his exposure to whatever it was on the floor that frightened him. My only consolation in watching Ray go through this routine was that he was still moving from one place to another. I knew that it was possible that if given enough time, OCD could convince him that it was too dangerous to walk on any surface and that it would be better for him just to stay in a few "safety" spots.

With every surface and object deemed contaminated, Ray found it impossible to find comfort in our home. He also couldn't touch anything without first pondering its recent history. Who had touched it last? When had they last washed their hands before they touched it? Could one of the cats have walked on it, causing it to become contaminated? Even doing something pleasurable, such as watching a movie, was dominated by OCD. Whenever Ray wanted to watch a movie, for example, he would first have to find a spot to sit on that felt right. With every chair, couch, and floor space deemed unacceptable, he would often watch movies perched on the edge of our fireplace hearth, and because it was parallel to where the television was, Ray would have to crane his neck just to see the screen. As for getting the movie started, Ray relied on me. With all that was swirling around in his mind, there was no way he could get the movie out of its case, into the VCR machine, and touch the buttons on the remote control without having to stop multiple times for hand washings.

Of all his avoidance strategies, the one that personally affected me the most was his aversion to human contact. Because he considered me contaminated, Ray couldn't stand to have me touch him. If I did, he would engage in a round of washing in a vain attempt to feel less anxious. During this time, I also couldn't hand him anything without him eyeing me like I was some sort of evil creature who was trying to harm him. And if our hands brushed, it was like my touch was a fire that had immediately burned him. He would flinch as if in pain, immediately withdraw his hand, and flee to the nearest sink to wash away whatever "filth" I had infected him with. At one point, Ray wouldn't even allow me to hand him things; he would insist that I put down whatever it was so that he could pick it up and not worry that we might accidently touch. At his worst, even this strategy wasn't good enough. If he even thought that I might have recently touched something that he needed to use, he would not pick it up. At dinner, for example, he would often use a napkin to pick up the fork he knew I had placed by his plate, carry it to the nearest sink, throw it in, and then get another one. I never pointed out to him that it was my hands that had put the forks in the drawer and that the one he now deemed as clean had been touched by me. I didn't want to give any more ideas to his OCD; it was very capable of generating enough on its own.

Ray also had another OCD-directed avoidance behavior. He didn't take care of his appearance. He was clean because his OCD demanded that he shower often, but he didn't do other things he should have, such as combing his hair, brushing his teeth, using deodorant, or caring about what clothes he wore. At a time when most teenagers

60

are concerned about how they look and are spending endless hours preening, Ray was stubbornly refusing to pay attention to his appearance. He had let his hair grow long, but because he didn't take care of it, it was a snarled mass. His clothes, like his body, were clean, but because he didn't pay attention to what he put on, he looked odd. OCD had caused all this to happen via one simple idea: Ray didn't want anyone to think he was attractive. His OCD had caused him to think that if he took care of how he looked, it meant that he was trying to sexually hurt another person. In Ray's OCD-twisted mind, he felt safer and more in control when he thought that he was ugly.

It was terrifying to watch as Ray's world continuously shrunk because of his OCD-induced avoidance. It was like watching the only light in a dark room gradually dim. What would happen when that light was completely extinguished (ie, when Ray's OCD closed out the entire world)? Would that mean that his life was over? After all, most life can't survive in complete darkness. Would it even be possible to rekindle the light? I knew that Ray was on a dangerous trajectory because of how his OCD was closing off his world. Sometimes, I think it was his OCD-induced avoidance that scared me the most. I hated his compulsions and the resources they took from him and his obsessions for hijacking his normal thinking, but the growing isolation that was occurring because of all his avoidance truly scared me.

Ray also thinks that his avoidance behaviors caused him much trouble and now realizes how OCD can cause one to become isolated.

ΔΔΔΔ

The number of things that triggered my OCD obsessions was small at first. When my OCD was in its infancy, touching only one door handle in the house would trigger my obsessions. To avoid that one handle was easy. In fact, avoiding that one door handle was so easy that none of us really worried about it. However, as more triggers arose, I was soon avoiding almost everything in my house.

At one point during my OCD, I was avoiding every doorknob out of fear of contamination. My rationale was that if someone had touched a doorknob that I knew was contaminated and then touched other doorknobs, it meant that all those other doorknobs were also contaminated. I also avoided touching my cats for that same reason. I avoided touching sink handles, eating utensils, walls, clothes, and even people. It got so bad that I retreated to the only place of relative safety: My room. I would go there and stay and anytime I ventured out, I was guaranteed anxiety and a set of uncontrollable compulsions.

The severity that my avoiding habits progressed to mirrored their negative effects on my life. The more I avoided things, the worse I got, and the more frustrated I became. For example, I was deathly afraid of touching the doorknob to my room since my mom had also touched it. Therefore, I used sheet after sheet of paper as barriers so I could turn the door handle. After a while, I ran out of paper and resorted to using my textbook pages for paper. There was a French textbook that I had borrowed from my school that I completely tore up to use as paper for opening doors. In addition, homework was frequently sacrificed for this same purpose and thus, my teachers would look down on me for not turning it in.

I would also only walk on certain paths on a floor that I felt were safe. There was a bathroom in my house that I was certain was contaminated. I felt that because my mom had walked on that bathroom floor and then walked on other floors that she had contaminated every floor in our home. Therefore, I would design intricate patterns of walking that I thought were safe. Watching me walk around my house must have looked ridiculous with me walking next to a wall for a couple steps and then jumping several feet to the next place where I felt was safe.

Another avoidance I remember well was avoiding any physical contact with people who had entered my house. I never touched my mom out of knowing that she had gone into the bathroom that I was scared of and had touched things in there. Without a doubt, this took a toll on her. Likely, it made her sad and made her question her efficacy as a parent. However, I remember trying to explain to her that I was afraid of her because of contamination and not because I did not like her.

Strangely, most of my avoidance behaviors centered on my home. I did have some at school and in other public places, but mostly they were at home. Thus, my home became associated with a place of immense stress and being at home was not something I wanted to do. My avoidance behaviors were only one part of my OCD, but they were very destructive to my social and family life. I could not have friends over to my house nor could I interact well with any person in my family who had been to my house.

Continuing Symptoms After Treatment

As with many who have OCD, Ray's symptoms didn't stay the same over time. Over the years and as a result of different types of treatments, Ray experienced an ever-changing array of symptoms. There were some that didn't change and stayed persistently with him, but there were others that withered away without us ever knowing why. Some symptoms simply morphed into new forms, and others appeared out of nowhere. The one thing, however, that stayed constant for a long time was the sexual nature of his symptoms.

After the onslaught of Ray's OCD symptoms, it was hard to imagine what additional aspects of sexuality that his OCD could latch onto and turn into obsessions. But unfortunately, Ray's OCD had a much more fertile imagination than mine and found new and creative ways by which to torture Ray. Even after he had started treatment (therapy and medication) and his symptoms had backed off, his OCD found new outlets. One new and distressing symptom that suddenly appeared was his obsession that an "emission" (ie, sexual secretion) might have occurred and that he had to "check" to see if it had. To do this, Ray would stop what he was doing and search for the nearest bathroom where he would examine his genital area. If his OCD detected the presence of any sexual material, which was often, Ray would engage in intensive washing or "confess" to me. If, however, a bathroom wasn't available or if time didn't permit him to perform his checking compulsion, then he would tell me that he was sure that he experienced an "emission" and that he was feeling bad about it. It took time, but I finally figured out that what Ray called an "emission" was probably, in many cases, a normal bodily sensation that we all often have. Whenever we are suddenly stressed, excited, or surprised we often feel a twinge in our lower abdomen. Ray's OCD had taught him to misinterpret these normal sensations as a sign of deviant sexual desires instead of normal, everyday feelings.

As Ray's treatment for OCD (ie, exposure and response prevention therapy) took effect, many of his smaller, less intense symptoms melted away even without being specifically targeted. It was as if when the main power source of his OCD was weakened, then its smaller outlets died away, much like when the trunk of a tree is cut and its branches no longer receive nutrients. In time, those branches die and fall off without ever having to be specifically cut away. With Ray's OCD, we saw this happening with several of his symptoms, such as being out in public with women present, touching certain surfaces in our home, walking on the floors in our home, petting our cats, and touching my hands. None of these symptoms had been focused on during Ray's therapy but still vanished as he progressed through his treatment. This observation was obviously a welcome surprise to me. When we had started his treatment, I assumed that every one of his symptoms would have to be singled out, targeted, and actively killed. It felt like we were expected to kill every single ant in a large anthill; I would do it if necessary to get Ray well again. But luckily, we didn't have to focus on every, minute OCD symptom.

Other symptoms, however, held on until they were specifically targeted and forced out of Ray's life. One small, but particularly annoying, OCD symptom that persisted in Ray was his extreme reaction when anything fell onto his lap. Because of his obsessions concerning sexual material, he would immediately deem anything that had fallen anywhere near his lap as contaminated, and it had to be either thrown away or cleaned. If the item was a piece of food, there was no problem, and I let Ray toss it away. If, however, the item was something more tangible, say a $20 bill or a credit card, then there was obviously a problem. Many times, he would refuse to let me have back whatever it was that had fallen on his lap without it being cleaned or without forcing me to wash my hands after handling it. Because I found this symptom so annoying and because it was not going away, I added it to the list of symptoms to be targeted, even though it wasn't one that caused him extreme problems.

A few of Ray's OCD symptoms were deemed unimportant enough to worry about and were incorporated into Ray's everyday existence. These were small enough not to affect his life in a substantial way and weren't ones that bothered anyone else. One of these symptoms was Ray's habit of pulling out his shirt so that it covered his lap, presumably as a way to protect the world from any wayward sexual secretion. With this habit, he would grab the front of his shirt, pull it out as far as it would go, and stretch it out over his lap. Anyone who saw him do this would probably think that his clothes were bothering him because they were scratchy or that he had some skin condition that caused his clothes to bother him. Even though I found this symptom annoying to watch and ended up buying him new shirts when his old ones had been stretched into disrepair, I let it go and hoped that one day he would stop doing it (he did).

Yet another category of OCD symptoms we encountered were those that had become habits even though the reason for doing them was no longer powerful. Long after Ray's OCD had been successfully treated and he was no longer bothered by his contamination obsessions, he would sometimes touch a doorknob in an unusual manner. Instead of using his whole hand to grasp the doorknob, he would twist it with his wrist like he was still afraid of contamination. Whenever I asked him why he did this and could he possibly grab the doorknob in a more normal manner, he often shrugged and then used his whole hand to open the door. Of course, I would then listen closely to see if he was washing his hands after touching the doorknob; maybe his OCD was still telling him to be wary and that he should wash up after encountering the doorknob. But, he never did. In time and with reminders (but not therapy), Ray stopped touching doorknobs in his unique way.

In retrospect, we realized that the driving force behind this particular behavior had stopped being OCD and had instead, become a habit.

OCD's Return After Therapy

I have often thought of OCD as an enemy who, even in defeat, would find ways to stay alive and attempt to rise again one day. I had hoped that this thinking was wrong and that I was being overly pessimistic. And, for a while after completing several rounds of therapy, it seemed possible that Ray's OCD was gone for good. His symptoms were negligible; he was regaining his confidence; and his outlook on life was healthy. But true to its nature, OCD found a way to invade Ray's mind once again. Even though I wasn't surprised by OCD's return, I was taken aback by one aspect: It took me a while to recognize it.

Even with all our accumulated knowledge and experience in dealing with OCD, it still managed to trick us and return to our midst for several weeks before we recognized its presence. It was like suddenly realizing that some despised person who we thought was dead was now sitting in our living room and had apparently been there for a while. How long had he (ie, OCD) been sitting there, and why didn't we see him come in? Did he come in through the door when our backs were turned, or did he somehow take some other form and sneak in? Who was supposed to be on guard, and why didn't they see his return and alert the rest of us?

There were several times during my dealings with OCD that I wondered if it was actually a living being who was intelligent, capable of learning (especially from its mistakes), and who could evolve to fit into changing environments. When Ray's OCD returned, it didn't come back in the same form as we had last seen it. It didn't make Ray obsess over sexual matters or convince him that the world around him was contaminated with sexual material. Instead, it hijacked one of Ray's hobbies and tried to take it over. Because OCD had camouflaged itself within a seemingly-normal and beneficial activity, we couldn't see it until it had done some damage.

During the last years of high school Ray had taken up physical fitness as a hobby. Like anyone who is discovering a new passion, Ray threw himself into this hobby. He read fitness magazines, researched the internet for information, joined a gym, and even bought some fitness equipment for home. Even though there were times when I wondered if Ray was thinking too much about his fitness, I didn't think it was a problem. After all, good physical health is a laudable goal, and he looked like he was having fun. It was only when he started talking about taking steroids that his new hobby became a problem. My first impulse to this idea was to tell Ray what I thought about steroids. Steroids were dangerous to one's health; the long-term effects of steroid use are unknown; and the purchase of steroids isn't even legal so it was too risky to try obtaining them. I had hoped that the totality of these arguments was strong enough to dissuade Ray from seriously thinking about taking steroids. But instead, he kept talking about steroids, arguing about their merits, and trying to find ways to obtain them. I, like an idiot, kept arguing back until one day, it struck me that these interactions caused me the same feelings of dread that his OCD once did. Whenever he came close to me, I dreaded it, suspecting that he would bring up steroids. He also looked anxious when he talked about wanting to take steroids, and he resumed having that far away look in his eyes that he often had when his OCD was in full force. He even progressed to the point where he would just look at me and say the word "steroids" without saying anything else.

Even though I had pledged to never again accommodate OCD, it forced my hand once again. The summer when Ray's OCD was focused on steroids was also a time when we planned to travel to Egypt. To get Ray even remotely excited about this trip, I had to address his OCD and make him some promises. Maybe I should have stood my ground and told his OCD what I really thought, but I didn't. I was afraid that if Ray's OCD didn't get what it wanted, then Ray might have refused to even go with us. How could I possibly enjoy such a fantastic trip knowing that my son was at home in the grips of OCD? So, I caved. I promised Ray that since steroids were legal in Egypt (a fact he had quickly found on the internet), we would look for them in some pharmacies. I also swore that we would find a fitness center every day we were gone so that he could maintain his routine. After he wrenched these promises from me, he reluctantly agreed to go with us but didn't appear happy about it. I suspected that he was a little suspicious of me, knowing that I was willing to boldly lie to his OCD.

Ray also realizes now, but not at the time, that his focus on fitness was also symptomatic of his OCD.

ΔΔΔΔ

During the summer between my junior and senior year of high school, my family and I planned a trip to Egypt. I was ecstatic, not because it was going to be such a fantastic trip, but because steroids are legal in Egypt (but not in the U.S.), and I was dying to get my hands on them. I had been working out for at least a year and was making good progress towards my bodybuilding goals, but I wanted even more progress. In fact, I had become obsessed over fitness and bodybuilding and not in a good way.

In a way, bodybuilding was helpful in dealing with OCD. Essentially, bodybuilding helped me mold a personality for myself, a personality that I had been desperate to form. By my junior year, I was the strongest kid in my class, and this gave me a strong sense of identity. Furthermore, bodybuilding gave me goals to work towards. It also enabled me to get excited about something and momentarily forget about the hassles of life. In other words, I always had something I could be proud of and help me feel like I was a successful person.

However, bodybuilding also became a source for my OCD to

70

latch onto and by the time we were to travel to Egypt, my obsessions over bodybuilding had spun out of control. I had made my mom incessantly promise me that while in Egypt, she would find a gym for me to workout at and a pharmacy where I could find steroids. (She never promised, however, that I could actually buy any.) I remember making her promise me hundreds of times to do this, and I even contemplated many times not going because I worried about not finding a gym. Any normal person would have immediately seen the benefits of traveling to Egypt and not worry so much over losing exercise time for a week. I, however, could not see those benefits and instead, I obsessed abnormally over the possibility of not getting to workout.

My steroid obsession even got to the point that I insisted on having my blood testosterone tested to make sure that my level was normal. I convinced my mother (and my psychiatrist who ordered the test) that the reason I wanted my testosterone level checked was because of my history of sexual obsessions and persistent feelings surrounding that issue. If I have told them the truth about my reasons for wanting the test, they would have never agreed to it. My hope for having the test was that if my level was low, then maybe I could get a prescription for steroids.

These bodybuilding obsessions were not easy to figure out. Using exposure and response prevention therapy or other techniques to treat this episode of OCD was hard because it might mean quitting exercise. This was not acceptable to me because I was also benefitting from the activity. My exercise was not only a compulsion but also something that helped me become more confident.

ΔΔΔΔ

Lucky for us, the trip to Egypt went well. We were so busy on most days that we dropped at night of exhaustion, and because of this frenetic pace, Ray didn't have the physical energy or mental focus to pursue his fitness. As for looking for steroids, he mentioned it occasionally, but because we didn't have control of our time and location, there wasn't much we could do about it, and by the end of the trip, Ray had stopped asking about steroids. In fact, he had stopped talking about them altogether. Why this happened wasn't clear, but it most likely resulted from his mind being so occupied with seeing such fantastic sites, such as the pyramids, the Nile, and ancient temples, that his OCD had found it hard to compete. Maybe because it had yet to fully reestablish itself in Ray's brain, his OCD hadn't had enough time to prepare itself for such an onslaught of competing stimuli. Whatever the reason was, it was clear that by the time we returned home, Ray's steroid obsessions had waned, and he was back to his baseline of minimal obsessions.

What our trip had taught me was that sometimes OCD can be pushed back in unexpected ways. By the time his steroid obsessions told hold, we were well versed in therapy for OCD and had spent countless hours in battling it. Based on our experience, I was preparing to fully engage it again once we returned home. I had already thought about what battle plan we would use, when we would start our offensive (ie, immediately), and was shoring up my mental reserves. When Ray's OCD retreated without much of a fight, I was floored. Here I was preparing for a full-scale onslaught, and my hated enemy had turned tail and run. Many times, I have wondered what role the trip played in pushing Ray's OCD back. Was it a coincidence, and it didn't have any effect at all? Maybe the same result would have occurred if we had stayed home. Or, did the change of environment somehow allow Ray's mind to ignore his OCD and give his normal functions a chance to regain their footing? Maybe the intensity of our trip, the constant moving about, and the barrage of new information was strong enough to short-circuit the OCD pathways.

I have never figured out why Ray's OCD remitted during this time, but it reminded me of an important lesson: OCD is unpredictable. Even those of us who routinely deal with OCD can never fully understand all its tricks; why it will dig in like a tic and refuse to relent during an episode but then inexplicably vanish during the next round. All we can do is to learn from each episode, try to find patterns, and continue looking for different weapons to use against it. Even though taking a long, expensive, and exhausting trip will never be the first idea I reach for when Ray's OCD flares up, I will certainly think about it.

Present OCD

It has now been several years since Ray's steroid and fitness obsessions threatened to derail his life. During this time his OCD has tried to return on several occasions, sometimes only managing to make itself known for about a day, but on other times, it formed into something more substantial and lingered for longer. None of these episodes, however, has remotely approached the intensity and duration that his sexual obsessions attained when he was younger. Needless to say, I hope that Ray's OCD never regains the force it once had and remains a shell of its former self. At this point, however, what I would like to know is the chance of that actually happening. Is the chance only 5% or is it closer to 80% that his OCD will one day return in full force and take over his life? No one can answer this question, of course; OCD is too diverse, and we are too individual-istic. Each of us who has dealt with OCD has developed different skills for dealing with it, has different support systems in place, and face different stressors in our lives. Trying to predict how OCD will behave for anyone who has it is like predicting what the weather will be in the next few years. It's not possible to do with any accura-cy. The best we can hope is for good weather on most days and for those days when the weather is bad, maybe even frightening, we can only hope that it passes quickly and doesn't cause much damage.

Even as Ray and I were writing this book, his OCD made an appearance. Within days of completing his finals at college, his OCD struck like lightning. There was no buildup to this episode; we had no hint that it was brewing. One day he was fine, happy, and relieved to be finally done with his classes, and the next, he was reeling with obsessions. The trigger for this episode was when Ray and his friend used some laboratory equipment at his university for a personal rea-son. Immediately afterwards, Ray started obsessing that he would be kicked out of school and that all his hard work at college would be for nothing. He worried that someone had seen them use the equipment and would question why they were in the laboratory. He incessantly worried about all this, even though no one had walked into the room while they were using the equipment. He worried that maybe someone had seen them through the window; maybe there was a hidden security camera in the room or the hallway that had recorded them; maybe they had left something in the laboratory that could be traced back to them; or maybe their fingerprints would be found. And, he compulsively contacted me for reassurance that he wouldn't be kicked out of school. Shortly after Ray first explained these worries to me, I knew: OCD was back. The bastard had returned.

What surprised both Ray and I about this episode was how quickly it appeared and loud it became. It was like OCD had its own version of shock and awe. It wasn't that we didn't expect it to return; in fact, I had reminded Ray that his semester breaks were a prime time for OCD to attempt a comeback and that he should keep a lookout for it. And, I was even more on guard for this break than I had been for previous ones. Ray's semester had been particularly tough; he had taken difficult classes, worked as a tutor for several hours each week, and had struggled to balance it all. His finals had also been hard, and he wasn't sure what grades he was going to receive. Added to all this stress was the worries that Ray had regarding his future. He couldn't decide what career path to choose and that uncertainly was weighing on him. My concerns during this time was that as soon as his finals were over and he no longer had a routine to follow, his OCD would march into the void, put down some roots, and try to grow. We knew this time would represent fertile ground for OCD and had prepared ourselves for its return.

I wish we could report that once Ray realized that his worries weren't real but were manifestations of his OCD that he got over it quickly and didn't have to struggle. Unfortunately, that's not what happened. For some reason, this episode was stickier than most and was stubbornly refusing to dislodge from Ray's brain. Initially, we had thought that this episode would behave like a similar one that had showed up during one of Ray's spring breaks. In that episode, Ray's obsessions lasted only about a day and were easily vanquished. All he did to get over that episode was to identify his worries as OCD, decide that he wasn't going to engage those worries, and refocus his thoughts away from his obsessions. It was amazing to witness. One moment he was reeling with OCD and the next, he was going out with friends and saying that his thoughts were no longer bothering him. After this episode, I had dared to hope that maybe OCD would never again take hold of Ray in a substantial way.

When Ray's latest OCD episode took hold we first tried using some simple maneuvers. No point tearing down a machine when the tightening of a few screws will solve the problem. Right? We identified the thoughts as OCD, cognitively evaluated the thoughts to show Ray they made little sense (a hallmark of OCD), and tried having Ray refocus his thoughts away from the obsessions. He was told to stay busy, to exercise daily, to go out with his friends, to not feed his obsessions by dwelling endlessly on them, and to not ask me for reassurance (ie, engaging in his compulsions). None of these ideas worked, and we quickly turned to exposure and response prevention therapy (ERP), the therapy that had helped us successfully deal with Ray's OCD in the past. The problem with this idea, however, was that it had been a long time since we used ERP and like any complicated skill, one loses their proficiency at it if they don't routinely practice. My first attempts at designing an ERP exercise for Ray failed, and he quickly lost patience with me. He made some attempts at it by himself but eventually declared that ERP couldn't work for him this time. I disagreed with him on this; I know how powerful

ERP is and have tried to convince him that the reason it was failing us now was because we hadn't worked on it hard enough. My instincts told me to stay with ERP, tinker with it until it worked, and then use it to beat this episode back. Ray remained unconvinced and because now he was older and more independent, I couldn't force him.

As these words are being written, Ray continues to deal with this latest OCD episode. It has relented some but is still too much alive for my comfort. We're not sure what caused it to fade but suspect several factors. For one, Ray has reestablished his routine at college; he goes to classes, tutors students in chemistry, and has started working in a research laboratory. These activities require mental effort which probably helps push out his unwanted obsessions. Ray also has started thinking about meditation and mindfulness as a way to deal with his worries and has so far, found these ideas helpful. I also, have not let up and have continued to challenge Ray's OCD in every way possible.

We are now certain that this most recent OCD episode will not be one that derails Ray's life. Its strength and tenacity, however, served to remind us that OCD is unpredictable and that if given a chance, it can reform and become an unstoppable force.

Part II – Understanding OCD

Introduction to Understanding OCD

I think that the worst enemies to have are those we can't see. Every day, we sense their threat, but they fail to take any real form. There's never a moment when they stand before us where we can confront them, shout at them, push them back, or do whatever it takes to make them leave us alone. And because they have no visible form, others around us can't see them. Even if we try to explain to others how our enemy is affecting us, sometimes even torturing us to the point of paralysis, they don't believe us. "I don't see anything to be afraid of," they tell us, "You're imagining all this. You just need to toughen up, grow up, and stop being so difficult. If you can't get over this, we will leave you behind and find someone more competent to spend our time with." What can we do then but to stop asking for help or even for validation? We are left alone to deal with our invisible enemy. If we're lucky, we might find some others who have similar enemies and who can help us find the right weapons to use or at least, give us hope that we are not as alone as we feel. In my life, I have dealt for many years with such an enemy and have had to help my son fight back the very same enemy: OCD.

OCD is invisible. Many times, I have wished that there was some way to make it more tangible, but as of yet, there isn't. There is no blood test, for example, to diagnosis and follow OCD, like blood glucose levels in diabetes, no imaging technique that can directly point to where OCD is, like tumors or infections, and no brain wave test to show the aberrant brain pathways that cause OCD, like EEGs do in cases of epilepsy. For those of us who have OCD, we have nothing to hold up to the world that proves our malady really exists, that it's as real as any physical affliction, and that we need help. I'm convinced that if we had something like a diagnostic test for OCD, then those of us who have it would seek out quicker treatment, suffer less derision from others, and would find our way back to health in much shorter times than what we currently do. As it stands today, many of us suffer quietly, afraid to speak of our pain because we worry that we will be stigmatized or worse, abandoned.

The experts tell us that they are closing in on what causes OCD and that someday soon we will have answers. What I hear in these promises is that they think that OCD will one day be made visible and as such, more easily explained. Instead of saying that those of us who have OCD have "something" wrong with our brain, we can say something more definitive like, "I have OCD because my caudate nucleus (a brain region) isn't functioning properly. This happened because I was born with too few dopamine (a neurotransmitter) receptors in that brain area." But, I doubt this will ever happen to such a level. The main reason for this thinking comes from the research that has already been done on OCD, especially that using brain scanners and gene probes. When people who have OCD are placed in brain scanners, for example, there are several areas that differ from those who don't have OCD. There has never been only one area that is involved, always several and even these appear to differ slightly between studies. And even with all this information, the experts still state that brain scanning shouldn't be used to diagnose OCD because the data remains too muddled for diagnosis. I wish this wasn't the case. I would love to have an MRI (or other brain scan) scan that shows where in Ray's brain it all went wrong. I would probably even request a copy to have on hand so that I could prove to those naysayers around us that Ray's symptoms come from a real brain disorder. "See, we aren't making it all up. Right here, this spot is why he has so many symptoms."

Without science or technology to help us, those of us who have OCD often struggle to define the condition that plagues us. We try, of course, but rarely succeed. Our barriers are many and come from varying sources. One problem, for example, that Ray and I have often stumbled over comes from how quickly others, who don't have OCD, think they understand it. Whenever we have tried to explain to others about OCD, we have often found that their first impulse was to search through their memories and find an example of their own obsessions. And when they remembered such an example (eg, a time when they were passionate or focused on something or someone), they would quickly declare to us that they understood all about OCD. To us, this was akin to someone visiting a Chinese restaurant and then declaring that they understood all there was to know about China and Chinese culture. Most times when this happened to us, we would try and patiently explain that having an obsession with someone or something was not OCD, but a normal, healthy, and desirable experience. But often, our words failed to dissuade our conversational partners from the idea that they understood OCD. Because they couldn't separate their own experiences from OCD, they failed to recognize OCD as the crippling illness it is. In other words, they refused to see us, the sufferers from OCD, as having a legitimate illness.

Until the time our condition is better understood, those of us who have OCD can help each other by telling our stories and striving to understand our condition. Through our stories and ideas about our OCD experiences, we can help those who continue to struggle to find their voices. We can, for example, tell our fellow sufferers of OCD how we have attempted to describe our OCD to others or explain other situations, such as the environments we grew up in, our current home life, or the struggles we face in the workplace, that we know has affected our OCD. Some of us have even had to deal with the guilt of passing our OCD onto our children and by explaining how we handled this emotion, we can help others who are wrestling with similar problems.

I encourage all who have OCD to talk, write, or blog about their OCD experiences. With our collective voices, I know that together, we can pull all who have OCD out of the OCD mud, get them cleaned off, and help them onto the road towards mental health.

Describing OCD

Even now, after all this time and experience in dealing with OCD I often fail to adequately describe what OCD is, especially to those who are naïve to its presence. Maybe this happens because OCD is complex and diverse in its presentation. OCD can manifest itself in many, different ways, which makes it hard to clearly state what OCD is and is not. A behavior, for example, that is helpful in one situation may actually be an OCD symptom in another. In other words, this monster can hide amongst us, using the veil of normalcy to avoid detection.

When asked to describe OCD, most people, especially those in the mental health profession, would probably use one of the official definitions of OCD, such as: *Obsessive compulsive disorder (OCD) is an anxiety disorder consisting of two symptoms, obsession and compulsion; although they are different, they are closely related and often occur in the same person. An obsession is a recurrent and persistent thought or desire. It is not voluntary and is distressing to the patient, but although the patient tries to suppress or ignore it, it is very difficult to eliminate from the mind. A compulsion is an uncontrollable urge to perform some repetitive and stereotyped action. This action is not an end in itself but serves as a substitute for unacceptable unconscious ideas and impulses. Although the patient does not know the reason for this action, failure to perform it leads to increasing anxiety, which can be relieved by giving in to the compulsion. Eventually, after repeatedly failing to resist the compulsion, the patient may lose the desire to resist it.*

This definition, and others like it, is informative, descriptive, useful, and necessary. (For the official description of OCD by the American Psychiatric Association please refer to the DSM-V, the bible of psychiatric diagnoses). For those professionals who study OCD, these definitions serve to clearly describe it. All these professionals have to do is to pull up one of these definitions, ask their patients a few questions, and decide: Does this person have OCD or not? But for those of us who have personally dealt with OCD, these textbook definitions don't relay the true colors of OCD. I would describe OCD rather differently.

One of the clearest words that I think describes OCD is pain. OCD is painful. Whenever an obsession would pass through my son's (Ray's) brain he would wince like he had just received an electric shock or had been stuck with a sharp object. Then, he would recover only to face the same jolt again and again. Sometimes, he would yell out in frustration after an obsession had jabbed him, getting angry that OCD was constantly attacking him, but at other times, he would stop, fall into the nearest chair and cry. And, there was little that I could do to help him. He was in constant pain, and for a long time, I had no way to lessen that pain.

Here's one of my attempts to describe what having OCD is like: OCD is like having to walk with a tack (ie, an obsession) in your shoe. Every step results in a sharp jab of pain. The effect of that tack, however, depends entirely on life's events. If, for example, you need to run from a burning building to save your life, you can ignore the tack and run as fast as you can. Your life is in danger, and you need to save it. The presence of something sharp in your shoe is not your primary concern. But, most moments in life are far removed from any drama. You need to get to school, work, and take care of your needs or the needs of your loved ones. The presence of a shoe tack in these moments will make itself known. Your mind registers pain during each step and in time, that pain takes its toll. You keep going, ignoring the pain and by the end of most days, you are exhausted and can't take another step. You often wonder why you have to deal with this constant pain, especially when you see how others go through their lives without limping (ie, without OCD). Perhaps you even give up, staying in bed because in bed, you don't have to walk and feel the pain of your ever-present tack. Also, when you look into your shoe you can't see anything sharp poking out of it, and when you show others your shoe and try to explain to them what is happening to you, they can't understand. They can't see anything in your shoe either and after a while, they start to chastise you for your constant limping. Some around you even think that you are faking it, trying to get away with something, and even suggest to you that you could stop limping if you would put your mind to it. (Other ways I have thought of to describe OCD include: Hitting yourself in the head with a hammer every fifteen seconds, holding a lighter to your fingertips several times per minute, or intermittently sticking a sharp object into an electrical socket. What these images share is the presence of pain that is repeatedly and endlessly felt.) Sometimes when I get frustrated by those around me who can't understand what having OCD is like, I think about hiding a tack in their shoe and making them walk on it for several miles. Then maybe, they would understand what those of us who have OCD experience.

Those of us who have OCD are in pain, a pain that is as real and crippling as any physical pain. But, we have yet to have that pain respected in many areas of our society. In any other medical situation, pain is assessed and then quickly addressed. You go into your physician's office with a sprained ankle, for example, and they ask you about pain; they will even want you to quantify it (on a scale of one to ten). Then, before you leave, you will receive instructions and medications to take that will alleviate your pain. This doesn't happen with OCD (or for other mental disorders). When we reach out to the medical professionals we are often told that we have to wait, sometimes for several months before they will even see us. What are we to do with our pain while we wait? We have no other choice but to bear it without relief.

Another problem that those of us who have OCD face when explaining OCD is that we often have to defend our disorder as real, medical, and life threatening. Imagine diabetics having to say things like, "I have diabetes because my pancreas no longer produces insulin. It's not because I ate all the wrong things and no, I won't be cured if I just stop eating doughnuts." Or, epileptics having to defend themselves by saying, "Please forgive me for having that seizure. I didn't want it to happen just then. I can't control it." Several times during Ray's OCD, I have had to explain that he can't control his symptoms, that he wasn't lazy and trying to get out of doing something, or that he could get over his "bad thoughts" if he really wanted to.

It's also often necessary for us to describe what OCD isn't. It's not, for example, about passions as in, "I'm so obsessed about my boyfriend. I think about him all the time and can't get him out of my mind." It's also not about achieving perfection as in, "I'm really obsessed about getting this job done right, or I'm so obsessed about my work that I can't think about anything else right now." And, it's not about being careful as in, "I'm obsessed about my family's safety so I double check to make sure our stove is off." Many of us who have OCD have had to deal with others who think they understand it and maybe even think that they have a "touch" of OCD. The one time that Ray and I told a school official about his OCD we ran right into this. Shortly after I mentioned Ray's condition, we were told by this official that he understood all about it; after all, he had to double check his door lock every night. I'm happy to say that I didn't yell or throw anything at him. I wanted to. I admit it. Instead, I forgave him for his ignorance, took a deep breath, and started explaining what OCD is and what it does to those who have it.

I use pain as a way of describing OCD to others. Ray, however, uses a different metaphor.

ΔΔΔΔ

When one of my friends asks me, "What is it like having OCD?," I often find myself in an uncomfortable situation. Understanding any mental illness, not just OCD, is a rare ability that generally only comes after direct experience with that mental illness. The perceptions that arise on television or in novels are often so inaccurate that those of us who do have a mental illness are overwhelmed with frustration and resentment at the media that both stigmatizes and overplays mental illness. When people hear "OCD," they think of their own behavior that remotely resembles OCD and may even exclaim, "I sometimes think I have OCD; I have to check that the door is locked twice every night." Or, they may think of people who are merely obsessive about their job or a hobby. So, where do I begin when trying to describe what OCD is really like?

I describe OCD by relating it to scenarios that everybody has gone through and that generates feelings that are akin to what someone with OCD would feel. One of the most pertinent examples I have thought of is to imagine the situation where you have a loved one who is in the hospital, bedridden, and is suffering from an illness that has only a 50% survival rate. Any free time that you have, you want to spend it with that person and whenever you are not with them, you worry about the possibility that the last time you saw them was the last time ever. Not an hour goes by without you being haunted by that possibility, and anything you do that normally feels good doesn't any more. Any success at work, for example, or receiving an A on a test that you had spend countless hours studying for could not be truly enjoyed because of the incessant worrying that you have about your loved one. You now live life below its fullest potential. Anything you previously felt as rewarding, such as hanging out with friends or going on a vacation, is now diminished by your constant worry. All aspects of your life are now meaningless because you constantly think about the fate of your loved one. And then finally, when it's all over, because your loved one has recovered and you try living your life as you used to, you are faced with the realization that you have missed so much because of the extent of your worrying. To me, the anxiety generated by OCD is equivalent to that of having a loved one in constant danger.

I have often thought that living with OCD is like always feeling a layer of anxiety above, beneath, and on the sides of all awake thought. In some sense, OCD acts as like a restraint around all thought, preventing new things from coming in and also preventing the expansion of your mind. Understandably, this description of OCD is an enigma to most, but I think it also accurately describes what it is like to live with OCD. Throughout their lives, anyone without OCD or other mental illness is open to try new things and learn new ideas. With OCD, however, every single step or action that is taken requires great deliberation. During my worst times of OCD, for example, I would avoid any situation that could stimulate my symptoms. Obviously, this behavior eliminated a huge amount of possibilities. I avoided hanging out with friends, participating in extracurricular activities in high school, petting my cats, and even, making conversation with people. Also, because of the complexity of my symptoms, I avoided almost any novel or strange situation that could possibly trigger my anxieties. All this resulted in my living life from a distance. Every thought I had that could be expanded into a creative endeavor or idea that could further me as a person was immediately diminished by a subsequent OCD thought.

What makes the experience even worse for a sufferer with OCD is the general lack of empathy among those who immediately surround them. When actions are actually the product of fear and anxiety induced by OCD (the compulsions), they are often mistaken for apathy or irritability. During my sophomore year of high school, for example, I had long, unkempt hair; my hands were red from so much washing; and my overall hygiene was poor. Because of my appearance, many of my classmates saw me as abnormal *and lazy. On occasion, I was verbally attacked with comments like "get a haircut." I was also never a favorite of my teachers. Several of my teachers did not like me because I was often late to class and often couldn't pay attention because of my OCD. It is understandable that these teachers assumed that my lateness was because I was being difficult, but in fact, it was all a product of my OCD.*

OCD and Genetics

One area of research that is actively involved in deciphering OCD's causes is genetics. Many researchers are currently searching through the human genome trying to find those genes that cause OCD. They're there, somewhere in our genes; that much is certain. Previous studies on OCD have proven that it runs in families, which means that its cause is partially genetic. In fact, it has been suggested that the cause of OCD is around 45%-65% genetic for those whose symptoms start in childhood. In other words, we inherit, through the genes our parents have given us, a good part of why we get OCD. I have often thought of this fact as a good news, bad news situation. Good news in that those of us who have OCD can point to a non-psychological cause for our OCD. "My OCD is caused by the genes I inherited and not because I am weak or lazy. I don't have OCD because I made mistakes in my life. I have it because of the bad luck I had when my genetic makeup was being formed." The bad news part, at least for me, comes from knowing that I gave my son his OCD. The guilt this knowledge brings has threatened to over-whelm me at times. Ray has suffered because of his OCD, and he has OCD because of me and my faulty genes. However, even with all this guilt I feel towards Ray, I have never harbored any ill will towards my mother, who most likely gave me those OCD genes.

Fortunate for me, Ray doesn't dwell too much on his un-lucky genetics. He has accepted his lousy luck in this area and has found ways to go on.

ΔΔΔΔ

During the worst times of my OCD, I would loathe my mom's side of the family because we are pretty sure that they had given me the gene (or genes) that made my OCD possible. I sometimes wish that I had been given a different set of genes that could enable me to forget about certain things that make me worry. However, this wishing has offered me no consolation, and I have realized that it is up to me to deal with it and find ways to have a good life.

Even though I may have been unlucky with regards to my genetics, I am lucky in one aspect: In my family, I am not alone in my fight against OCD. My mom has spent a majority of her life fighting OCD both in herself and in me. In a way, knowing that my mom has dealt with OCD in the same way I have offers me great comfort. Not only does it soothe me in knowing that someone else has gone through OCD the way I have, but it also gives my mom great credibility in terms of OCD treatment. I know that she understands how bad I really feel, maybe even better than any psychologist who has not directly experienced OCD. Thus, when she tells me about a way to think about OCD that helped her deal with hers, I am much more willing to give that way of thinking a try.

Unfortunately, we cannot control the genes that we pass to our children. Nor can we choose to keep or discard the genes that have been given to us. It is my duty to make the best of what I have and accept the faults with the good. I have found that if I waste too much time thinking about what I would rather have had or a route in life I wish I could have taken, I miss out on too much that goes on.

One of the greatest challenges in dealing with OCD is learning to accept certain thoughts that run through my head. I have also found that I can use this method of acceptance to help me get over any anger for being given such a horrible mental disorder.

ΔΔΔΔ

Even with all the work that has been done on OCD and its

genetics, the story is far from complete. No one has yet uncovered "the OCD gene" that definitively explains why OCD happens, and it's highly unlikely that such a gene even exists. Like many physical disorders (eg, heart disease, stroke, or cancer), OCD doesn't arise because of one gene that goes wayward but because of different genes that fail to function normally. As of today, many genes have been found that travel with OCD, and it's likely that even more genes will be identified as more researchers join the hunt. Not surprisingly, the genes that have already been discovered in association with OCD are all involved in brain function and direct such complicated functions as transporting neurotransmitters (eg, serotonin and dopamine) between brain cells, serving as receptors for neurotransmitters (eg, dopamine and glutamate), and acting as neurotransmitter brakes (ie, enzymes that breakdown neurotransmitters and stop their functioning). And, I'm sure that in time, other genes that direct other neurological activities will be implicated in causing OCD.

The main conclusion that I have come to after thinking about genes and OCD is simple: There are a lot of different genetic causes for OCD. Many, different roads get us there, not just one. It's not like there's one superhighway that funnels all of us towards OCD land. There are many ways to get there, some direct and fast and others more winding and slow. Some of us have genes that make us feel our OCD when we're kids and others have ones that keep our OCD at bay until adulthood. But even though we have all traveled different roads to get there, we have all landed in the same destination: A place where we never wanted to go and one in which we all strive to leave as soon as we possibly can. And once left, a place we never want to visit again.

In our family, we have three generations who have sported some OCD genes. I suspect that there were others in previous generations, but we will never know. Many times, I have wondered how old our OCD genes are or those of our fellow sufferers of OCD. No one can yet answer this question, but I bet that if researchers would someday search through the ancient genetic material of our prehistoric hominids, they would likely find the genes associated with OCD already in place. I can certainly imagine a cave man or woman endlessly obsessing and compulsing over their worries. "I just hit Org over the head with my club. Does that make me bad? I just gave my baby that red berry that we eat all the time, but how I do know for sure I didn't just kill him?" I also wouldn't be surprised if these same genes are active in our fellow creatures, in both those who are evolutionarily close to us, like chimps or gorillas, and in those that are more distant, like cats and dogs. In fact, some researchers have already described an OCD-like condition in some dogs (these poor creatures compulsively lick themselves raw) and in some rodents, who compulsively groom themselves. Since there are no ways to ask these animals about their thoughts, we don't know if they are having obsessions like we do. But, their compulsive behaviors look uncomfortably familiar.

Even though we don't know how old our OCD genes are, there is one fact we are sure of: These genes have been around a long time, maybe even as long as the written word. The ancient Greeks, for example, have left us records describing individuals who suspiciously sound like they suffered from OCD. But, this raises a question. Why have these genes lasted so long? One would think that genes that cause us so much pain and trouble would have died out long ago. After all, wouldn't it have been impossible to conceive and raise children during all the ravages of famines, wars, and diseases of our past if one's brain was stuck on the endless obsessions that OCD causes? In other words, how did our OCD ancestors survive? The only way this makes sense to me is to admit something that I loathe to do: Having OCD is good. Maybe our OCD ancestors were valued in their societies because they contributed in useful and unique ways. Maybe because they obsessed over cleanliness, always washing their hands, food, and children, they survived when others died of diseases. Perhaps their constant need for reassurance about food safety kept themselves and their friends from eating the wrong berries and dying. I can even imagine a scenario where obsessing over something as simple as whether a rock is really a rock and not a crouching lion is helpful for survival. Is it possible that our ancestors were actually the heroes, sages, and the wells of wisdom in their societies and were the ones everyone else turned to for guidance? And, because of the harsh environments they lived in, they didn't get stuck on their obsessions or compulsions like we do today. Their brains had to move on to other thoughts if they were to survive. Maybe those who have OCD are really saviors and kings that have been misplaced in time. Anyway, it's fun to think about.

Because OCD runs so strongly in our family, I asked Ray what he thought about it and whether our genetic heritage would make him hesitate about having children of his own. He is currently nineteen, and it's likely that his thinking on this will evolve as he progresses through life.

ΔΔΔΔ

OCD is hereditary, and if I ever choose to have children, they have a good chance (some sources say over 50%) of getting OCD from me. Because of this, I think it is most likely that I will never have children of direct descent. There are many reasons for my choice, and I understand that others in my situation would make a different decision. Giving life is incredible, but I wonder if it might not be ethical for me impart it if I know that severe suffering is possible and probably likely. If my children ever had to deal with OCD the way I have, I would feel guilty to point that I could not bear it. I would also worry about the possibility that the person I gave OCD to might not be able to take care of themselves if for some reason, I was no longer around. I realize that some may argue that because of my extensive experience in dealing with OCD that I would have the necessary skills to help my children through it, but I still don't think that passing along my OCD is a risk I want to take.

Despite my hesitations to have any children of direct descent, I still want to have them in my life. I plan take care of some children whether it is through adoption or they being the children of someone in my life. Going through life without having children seems too lonely. I also want to experience that kind of love that can only be felt by parents towards their children, and I don't want to have that love be missing from my life. I hope also to someday feel that I have a vastness of knowledge and experience that I want to impart onto somebody and who better to have around during that time than a child?

Despite my personal opinions on having children, I do not mean to say that someone with OCD should never have their own kids. If a person with OCD is okay with taking those chances of passing along their OCD, then by all means, they should go for it. It can be argued that giving life is better than not giving it at all out of fear of possible OCD. After all, life is truly the ultimate gift.

A situation that got me thinking about children and the risks we take bringing them into this world occurred on a television series where the main characters had to live in a world that was populated with zombies that threatened to kill them. One of the women in the show was pregnant, and the group she lived with had to decide whether or not it was ethical to bring a child into a world that was filled with such suffering. After a long discussion, they decided that it was worth having that child. The parents knew that they would have nothing but unconditional love for that child. They knew from experience that unconditional love from another human being trumps all other discomforts in life. With such love, a person knows that they are *never alone and that someone is there to look out for them.   This is the type of love that can overcome all life's difficulties, including OCD.*

OCD and Environment

OCD isn't explained solely on the presence or absence of one or more genes. It's not that simple. Genes are also affected by the environments in which they land. In other words, the same constellation of genes that might cause OCD in one person could fail to do so in another, all because we live in different environments. This idea, of course, isn't unique to OCD but is commonly seen in many conditions. Someone may, for example, have genes that predispose them to heart disease and if they smoke, spend most of their time sitting, and eat a high-fat, cholesterol-laden diet, then chances are, they will have heart disease and will probably suffer several heart attacks. This same person, however, could possibly avoid having heart disease if they refrain from smoking, exercise often, and eat carefully. If fact, they might not even know that they are at risk for heart disease because they have directed their life in such a manner that kept their heart safe. For heart disease and for many other conditions, our genes are not entirely in control. To understand the entire story, we also need to consider our environments.

With OCD, it's not easy to determine what environments cause us harm and what ones protect us. It's too complicated. I wish it was as easy as eating more fruits and vegetables and increasing exercise like it's for lessening heart disease, but it's not. No one can say what environments allow OCD to brew and which ones keep it at bay. In fact, those who have OCD have popped out of every environment: High income, low income, highly educated, poorly educated, religious, agnostic, urbanized, or countrified. In addition, OCD has been found in every culture where it has been looked for. All environments, regardless of location or resources, are capable of germinating and supporting OCD.

In lieu of finding the perfect environment for the prevention of OCD, we can instead, strive to live in environments that are conducive to good mental health in general. No one does well, for example, in environments where there is a lot of yelling, hitting, neglecting, ignoring, or criticizing. Even those whose genes are free from the susceptibility of mental illness can't thrive in homes that are full of negativity. They would, however, do better than those of us whose genetics predispose us to mental disorders. They would have more resilience and flexibility in their thinking, and they could use those abilities to help them survive. In other words, they would have more routes of escape available to them.

I have often wondered if I had done something that caused Ray's OCD to flare. Maybe some aspect of our home environment that I had created was responsible for sparking Ray's OCD and had I been a better parent then he wouldn't have gone through his OCD hell. If I had been smarter, less self-absorbed, and more attentive, then maybe he could have been spared the worst of his OCD storm. I will never know for sure and have finally, stopped beating myself up over this idea. But, I have also concluded that there were areas where I could have done better and in doing so, may have saved Ray some anguish. I have always, for example, regretted the intensity that routinely ran through our home. I was a busy, small town pediatrician who was often called away in the evenings, weekends, and holidays to take care of patients and who also had the type of OCD which demanded perfection. Needless to say, I was usually tense, focused on my patients, and quick to dismiss any questions or concerns that Ray might have. I know that he sensed this intensity and that it probably caused him to feel insecure. After all, how safe can a kid feel if he knows that every time he makes a mistake or has a problem, his mother will only sigh, frown, shake her head, or even yell at him? Instead of calmly asking questions and trying to find a solution, I would often be quick in my answers to him and dismissive of his worries. I suspect that if Ray had felt more secure, then his OCD would have had a harder time finding ground. OCD thrives in stressful environments, and an intense home is undeniably a source of stress.

Even though a stressful home environment isn't ideal for preventing OCD, it's not solely responsible for sparking OCD. In many OCD memoirs, the authors describe growing up in a loving and calm home and can't see any link between how they were raised and their OCD. In these cases, familial stress was nonexistent and therefore, wasn't a contributing factor to sparking OCD. Other memoirs, however, describe home environments where intensity, criticism, and high expectations were all present. But even in these memoirs, the authors don't describe a direct connection between their OCD and how they were raised. In other words, they don't blame their parents for their OCD, but instead, suggest that their homes could have been more peaceful. Even though it's difficult to directly link OCD with a stressful home environment, there are enough hints to suggest that lessening the noise, turmoil, and upheaval in one's home might help.

In addition to living in a less intense home, Ray also could have used a more attentive one. Ray was never neglected, of course; he was fed, talked to, ferried wherever he needed to go, and taken to different places. What he didn't have, however, was time with me where we could just be. We rarely had time where we could talk to each other or decide at a moment's notice what we wanted to do. When we were together, I was usually the one deciding what to do, where to go, and when we had to get back home. Because of this approach, I didn't know Ray very well. I assumed that I did, but I realize now that most times, I was talking at him and not with him. If I had the opportunity to go back in time and redo anything I wanted, one of the first things I would change was how I spent my time with Ray. Instead of always pushing towards some goal, I would stop and make a space where he could create whatever he wanted. I would sit in that space with him, quietly watching him, helping him only when he asked for it, and watching to see what he made. In other words, I would give him my undivided attention whenever we entered this space. I also wouldn't judge anything that came out of that space, but would instead, learn from it because it would tell me something important about Ray and who he is.

If Ray and I had routinely spent time together in our personal space, then I suspect that OCD would have had a much harder time digging in. I would have seen it coming on because I was watching Ray and would have realized much quicker that what Ray was saying and thinking was unusual for him and that something was brewing. This awareness, had it happened however, doesn't mean that we would have immediately known what to do, but it would have given us some time to learn about OCD, ask questions, and find the best plan of action. What happened instead was that I assumed that what Ray was experiencing was benign. I also didn't want to think about it being something more serious. After all, I didn't have time for dealing with a mental illness, and it was much easier to pretend that Ray was going through a normal developmental stage than it was to consider that he was showing signs of OCD. Because of this blindness on my part, Ray's OCD got worse than it might have, which made it much harder to treat. It's like the difference between digging oneself out of debt when only about $1,000 behind as opposed to $100,000.

One of the reasons that I failed to provide Ray with an environment that might have protected him from OCD was because of something we all face: Competitiveness. In today's society, we are expected to compete, work long hours, sleep less, and sacrifice our family time if we want to succeed. I had fallen right into this thinking. I was physician and had spent years working long hours because I assumed that I had to; otherwise, I would be deemed as less successful. Why so many of us have to live in this dog eat dog, sacrificial, elbowing, stomping world of ours is not something I understand. How did we get here, and why did we let it happen? And, how the hell can we stop it? I can't see how this stressful world is good for any of us, but for those of us with OCD (and sufferers of other mental disorders) it only adds to our problems. If someone has to start their day fighting off their internal demons, how can they possibly handle the additional ones that lurk outside their doors? I don't have any solutions for this dilemma. It would take someone far wiser than me to change the world in such a dramatic way. But what I can do, however, is to encourage my fellow sufferers of OCD to guard against getting sucked too far into this world. I doubt that any of us can avoid it altogether, but maybe we can control how far we fall. If, for example, our school or work place is fraught with stress and competitiveness, we should focus on making our home life as peaceful and nurturing as possible. We should also protect our downtime and do only those things that relax us and spend our time with those who allow us the freedom to be ourselves. In other words, we need to ignore the constant messages we hear from others and learn to live on our own terms.

Whenever I think about our environments and the difference they make in our lives, I'm reminded of a story of a woman who has OCD and schizoaffective disorder (a mental condition where someone has elements of schizophrenia, like delusions, and mood problems, such as depression). She struggled terribly for years, was unable to hold a job, and was hospitalized for her symptoms on several occasions. She received treatment but still couldn't keep a job until she was lucky enough to find an organization that was willing to help folks like her. She was given a job in the mental health arena but was also given something else: An environment that didn't shun her. She was surrounded by colleagues who understood and accepted mental illness and were willing to give her what she needed. Sometimes these things were simple, like reassurance. When she would say something like, "Did you just hear that voice saying something (a common symptom in schizophrenia)?," her colleagues would simply say "No," and she would then know to ignore that voice and go on with her day. Imagine what would happen in any other work environment if someone said something like that. They probably wouldn't have their job for long. On occasion, this woman also needed and received additional benefits. If she felt her anxiety spinning out of control, she was allowed to take time off and regain her balance without worrying about losing her job. Also (and this is my favorite part of the story), she was allowed to bring a dog, who had been specifically trained to help people deal with their anxiety, to work whenever she needed it. Amazingly, this dog would also often comfort others (by snuggling up to them) in the workplace because he sensed they also needed his help. This work environment allowed this woman to remain active, contributing, and most importantly, mentally healthy. Why can't we all have such places to work, study, or simply, live?

Ironically, there is one exception to this goal of living in a nurturing and calm environment that pertains particularly to OCD. When we need to undergo treatment with exposure and response prevention therapy (ERP), we need other, more unconventional aspects to our environment. OCD causes us such havoc that to effectively deal with it, we often have to use unique tools and be willing to temporarily exist in environments that others might shun or that might harm us in other situations (for those readers who are skipping around, please refer to the chapters on ERP if needed to understand this idea). In other words, we might have to temporarily sacrifice our attempts at a peaceful, quiet, and nurturing home and exchange it for a mini battlefield full of explosions, smoke, and intense yelling. When Ray was undergoing ERP, I realized that to be successful at it, we would need intensity, brute force, and dictator-like leadership from me. If anyone had seen our home during the time we were actively taking on OCD, they would have turned and run thinking that we had lost all sense. But for what we need-ed to accomplish, this was exactly the environment we needed.

Like me, Ray can't pinpoint any particular aspect of our home environment that directly caused his OCD, but he does have a few ideas about how OCD might have gotten a stronghold in his life.

ΔΔΔΔ

I have always wondered about the circumstances that pushed me to develop full-fledged OCD. Professionals say that there is a combination between nature and nurture that help to mold a person's persona, but I have only successfully identified the nature component. I know that my mom's side of the family has OCD, and OCD being hereditary, it was passed to me. But, I have always wondered about the nurture component. In other words, what in my environment pushed me to develop OCD?

I have no memory of instances of abuse, shock, or immense fear that made me develop OCD, especially my sexual obsessions. If I had been sexually abused or sexually traumatized in any way, I could see how OCD could easily latch onto sexual obsessions because I would already be sensitive in that area. However, I was not abused in any way which has always made me wonder why OCD chose sexuality as its topic.

One idea I have about why OCD affected me so much is loneliness. In other words, was I too lonely as a child? Did I spend too much time by myself with nothing but the company of my own thoughts? When I think back to my childhood, this seems likely to be a contributing factor. Because my mom was busy as a physi-cian, I spent a majority of my after school and evening time at home playing computer games rather than building up myself through academics, social gatherings, or through hobbies. In fact, even now I often feel as if I do not have many skills or talents be-

104

cause I have spent too much time doing things that did not contribute to building a good sense of self identity and security. My mom disagrees with this idea, of course, but I still think about it at times.

Could this lack of identity contribute to how my OCD affected me and how drastically it affected me? It is hard to say but intuitively, it makes sense. When OCD began creeping up on me, I didn't feel as if I had many positive elements to fight it back with. If I had been a painter, for example, who loved nothing more than to paint, maybe I could have used that to reach goals and override my OCD. Or, if I had been more musically inclined, I could have used that. In other words, if I had found something that I could have been working on all along and that allowed me to build an identity, then maybe OCD wouldn't have found such an easy way into my life.

I also wish that I had been more social when I was younger. I had always found it hard to communicate well with others, and in many ways I'm still a little shy. I have always wondered that if I had been more outgoing and surrounded by good friends, then maybe my OCD wouldn't have gotten so intense. I will never know for sure, but it's something I think about on occasion.

OCD and Comorbid Conditions

Further complicating our understanding of what causes OCD is another observation: OCD often doesn't travel alone. In other words, many of us (perhaps as high as two thirds) who have OCD also have additional diagnoses. In fact, the list of possible comorbid conditions is long and includes such diagnoses as major depression, attention deficit hyperactivity disorder (ADHD), general anxiety disorder, Tourette's syndrome, panic disorder, and phobias. Less commonly, diagnoses, such as bipolar disorder, schizophrenia, impulse control disorders, trichotillomania (ie, compulsive hair pulling), body dysmorphic/eating disorders (eg, anorexia and bulimia nervosa) can also coexist with OCD. In fact, I wouldn't be surprised if every mental condition that has ever been described has been co-diagnosed with OCD in at least one person.

Why mental disorders often travel together isn't clear. Maybe the brain pathways that are affected in multiple disorders lie in so close proximity to each other that whatever causes one disorder also sets off the others. In other words, whatever is responsible for causing a mental illness acts not with a surgical precision but more like a bomb that affects a wide swath of territory. Another idea is that the symptoms of one disorder so affects a person's life that eventually, symptoms of additional problems start to take hold. The addiction disorders, like drug or alcohol abuse, often follow in the footsteps of other disorders. It's easy to understand, for example, how someone with OCD could resort to using drugs or alcohol just to get a modicum of relief. It's also not surprising that major depression is often diagnosed after someone has been dealing with OCD for years. What could possibility be more depressing than the constant pain and loss that OCD causes?

Another possibility as to why mental conditions are often diagnosed together is that the professionals, who are making the diagnoses, are making mistakes and are incorrectly attributing certain

OCD symptoms to the wrong disorders. Ray's OCD, for example, often caused him to be inattentive in the classroom and if these symptoms had been brought up during an evaluation, it's likely that he would have been diagnosed with ADHD and prescribed a medication, such as Ritalin or Adderal. There were also many times when Ray's OCD forced him to defy his teachers and other authority figures, and it would have been easy to apply the diagnosis of oppositional defiant disorder to him. And, I have no doubt that if a mental health professional was watching Ray when his OCD had caused a major meltdown and he was raging, complete with yelling, stomping, whirling, and flinging, that they could have pointed to the page in their books and showed me how he was meeting the criteria for rage attacks and suggest that we give him yet another medication like Xanax (a benzodiazepine like Valium or Ativan that is often used to calm people down).

In Ray's case, we focused on treating the OCD and waited to see what would happen to his other problems of inattention, defiance, and anger outbursts. In fact, I never mentioned these problems to any of the mental health professionals we consulted. My reason for taking this approach was not because these other symptoms weren't significant (they were), but because I worried that Ray might be prescribed medications that specifically targeted these symptoms. Even though I am not opposed to using medications for mental illnesses (Ray took some), I was not willing to have Ray on more than one medication at a time unless it was absolutely necessary. If Ray had been taking several medicines at once, (eg, Zoloft for his OCD, Ritalin for his inattention, and Xanax for his rages), then it would have been difficult to determine which ones were helping what symptoms and how to make adjustments for continued symptoms. If, for example, Ray had had increased problems with paying attention, should we have increased his ADHD or his OCD medication? My other concern was that I didn't want Ray to think that medications were the only answers to his problems. In many cases, this thinking wouldn't be wrong; medication has brought miracles for many who are suffering. But for OCD, other therapies (ie, exposure and response prevention therapy) are more effective than medications even though they are difficult to undergo. If Ray had learned to always turn to medications for his problems, I worried that he might have refused to push through his therapy. He might have sat down, refused to even try, and demand that I find another pill to help him.

We were lucky. As Ray's OCD was improving, his other problems were also retreating. In fact, once his OCD was pushed so far back that he no longer met its criteria, most of his other problems had also vanished. He could pay attention in class and no longer experienced episodes of rage. But even with this amazing progress, there remained one problem that refused to budge: A depression. And not only did it refuse to lessen, there were times when it loomed larger. This probably happened because the depression had been masked by the largeness of Ray's OCD, and once that OCD was waning, the depression now had room to grow. I was dismayed and a little surprised by Ray's depression but really shouldn't have been. He had gone through so much with both his OCD and its treatment that it made sense that his mind had wound down and was now refusing to move on until it got time to rest and recuperate.

Of all the additional conditions that affect those of us who have OCD, the one that occurs most often is depression. It has been estimated that up to two thirds of those with OCD will also have to deal with depression at one or more times during their lifetimes. This marked degree of depression isn't surprising when we consider how OCD wears us down, every day, sometimes for years on end. And then, when we do decide to reach for help, we are often disappointed by what we find. Maybe OCD destroys so much in us that we give up trying to live, a situation which then leads us directly into depression. The good news is, however, that the depression that accompanies OCD isn't unique or more resistant to therapy than that depression which affects others. It's treatable with medications and with talk therapy. In fact, for those of us with OCD, receiving treatment for depression is easier than undergoing the therapy for our OCD.

In time, Ray's depression waned. It still shows up on occasion and causes him some trouble but never lingers for too long. He pushes through his negative feelings and finds a way to move on with his life. I suspect that, like his OCD, depression will return on occasion but will not take over his life. Ray, however, sees his depression as much more troublesome and currently thinks that its effects run deeper than his OCD. The reasons for our differing views on this aren't clear, but I suspect that it has something to do with how we remember Ray's OCD episodes and his current stage in life. I vividly remember each OCD episode and the pain it caused, whereas Ray often doesn't. Also, he currently feels the stresses and depression that many college students feel at this stage of their lives. The endless classes, the uncertainty of future prospects, and the competition for reaching the next step are all things that cause anxiety and depression even in those who have no history of mental disorders.

ΔΔΔΔ

By nature, I am a pessimist. I cannot help but see the faults and uncertainties in most people I meet and in most new situations I find myself in. When it comes time to take a new class, for example, I often find that I am sighing in anxiety and searching for ways to get an A in the class and not looking at the class as an opportunity to learn. Because of the way I am, I get quickly stressed and thus, get depressed easily. Sometimes this depression can hit me so hard that each day becomes a burden and is hard to get through.

Over one summer I became obsessed with the idea that because I was not getting enough sleep, I would never become the great scientist or doctor that I aspire to be. I worried incessantly about my sleep to the point we realized that it was probably a symptom of my OCD. But there was a difference between these thoughts and my previous OCD symptoms: These new thoughts caused me to feel very depressed. Many times, I sank into a chair while my mind slowly accepted the idea that I would never reach the potential my family and friends thought I could. I even decided that I will always be a failure. These thoughts plunged me into a depression like I had never felt before when fighting my OCD-related sexual thoughts. With those thoughts I felt pure anxiety but never real depression.

There are times when I think the pain of depression outweighs the pain I felt with my OCD symptoms. To me, there were times when my depression seemed endless. I would try, each day, to pull myself out of a depression only to find that on the next day that it was still there and was seemingly as strong as ever.

The ways I found to deal with these depressive thoughts consisted of two things: Friends and meditation. Whenever I went to spend time with friends, I could quickly pull myself out of a depression. I became social; I thought things were funny; and I looked at every situation with positivity. I could even come home afterwards and still feel good for several hours before I started to slump back into my negative thoughts. The other answer that I have just recently discovered is meditation. Now whenever I feel low, I focus all of my attention onto the silence around me or the stillness of my body and within about ten minutes, I feel better. Through meditation, I can relax in almost any situation and free myself of anxiety and sadness.

Sexual Obsessions

OCD comes in many different flavors. There is the vanilla (ie, the most common) of OCD: The germaphobes who obsess over "dirt" and who compulsively wash their hands and bodies. Then, there are the chocolate and strawberry forms of OCD, who consist of checkers, counters, and confessors. These common flavors (types) are so frequently discussed in OCD books or portrayed in the media that they now represent "normal" OCD, that is, the types that most people think of when considering OCD. Many times, I have wished that Ray's OCD had taken one of these more common forms instead of sexuality. It's bad enough to have an uncommon condition (OCD affects 1%-2% of the population), but to have it assume one of its more uncommon forms is like adding insult to injury.

Thanks to modern media, many people have now heard of OCD. News programs, talk shows, and radio programs have all had their segments on OCD where they talk to authors of OCD books, people who suffer from OCD, and the mental health professionals who treat it. There is even a TV series where each week, someone who has OCD is spotlighted, and the audience watches their treatment process. I am thankful for all these efforts. Because of them, OCD is now better understood among the populace and is more accepted as a legitimate condition that deserves attention and treatment. But, I do have one complaint against all this attention: Nobody talks about sexual obsessions. It seems that those who have sexual obsessions are like the ugly stepsister who is kept in the attic. She exists, but no one wants the world to see her.

I watch every media segment I can find on OCD, from the major networks to the smaller, local ones, hoping that one will show someone with OCD whose OCD focuses on sexuality and what they did to deal with it. But, I have yet to find one. Why this topic isn't addressed isn't clear to me, but several ideas leap to mind. Maybe those who have sexual obsessions refuse to publicly identify themselves, or maybe the networks are too timid to discuss sexuality in such a dramatic and confusing way, fearing that their audience will take offense. Perhaps the producers of such programs fail to educate themselves on sexual obsessions and think that those who have such thoughts are dangerous sexual predators or pedophiles and don't really have OCD. I hope that sometime soon, all these reasons for not addressing sexual obsessions are overcome and some brave souls are allowed to talk about their experience. Who knows, maybe it will be Ray who finally breaks the ice.

Many books on OCD mention sexuality as one form that OCD can assume, but they rarely give this topic much individual attention and often throw it in the same group as violent obsessions. Even the annual conference that is held by the International OCD Foundation doesn't have many sessions discussing what to do about sexual obsessions. It's hard to figure out why the experts don't think that it's important to give sexual obsessions more focus; maybe they think that someone who has these obsessions can get enough information about their OCD without being specifically exposed to their subtype. Maybe I'm the one who's wrong and that the topic of sexual obsessions really is adequately covered in the OCD books. My bias, of course, is that the available information on this topic is not nearly enough. If it were up to me, I would have the OCD experts write at least one book that was solely dedicated to discussing sexual obsessions and how to treat them.

Because Ray's OCD focused on all aspects of sexuality, we looked far and wide for any information on sexual obsessions that would help us. We wanted to know, for example, how common is sexual obsessions in OCD; what are the reasons why some who have OCD focus on sexuality; and how does one treat sexual obsessions? Most of the information we found was too general or vague to help us, an observation that only served to demoralize us even more. After all, if even the experts can't or won't talk about sexual obsessions in a detailed way, what does that say about us? Finally, after some digging, we found one book (*The Imp of the Mind*, by Lee Baer) that helped answer some of our questions. After reading this book, we no longer felt alone. There really were others who, like Ray, suffered from sexual obsessions and who had found ways to overcome their bad thoughts.

When Ray was struggling with his sexual obsessions, we told no one. We feared that others wouldn't understand and might even mistake Ray for a sexual deviant. I advised Ray to not talk about it with anyone, particularly his teachers or his parent's friends. One of my recurring nightmares during that time was opening my door to find child protective services standing there demanding information regarding my son's focus on sexual matters. I feared that some teacher or other mandated reporter would call the authorities because they failed to understand that Ray's worries stemmed from OCD and not because he had been sexually abused. I even had imagined what Ray might have said if he had been questioned during this time. I doubt whether he would have told anyone that he had OCD and that his focus on sexual matters was a result of this mental disorder. I suspect that he might have just sat there, staring at the floor, unable to answer the barrage of questions coming at him. Maybe I was paranoid, but I could see how Ray might be taken away from me because of someone's ignorance of OCD.

After Ray's OCD had improved, we tried explaining to others what he had gone through but soon gave up. On several occasions when we mentioned that Ray's OCD had focused on sexual matters we were asked, "Does that mean he wants it (ie, sex) all the time?" "No," we would patiently explain, "it doesn't. He doesn't have a sexual addiction. That's a whole different problem. Sexual obsessions in OCD have nothing to do with desire, but with fear." We would often be met with a puzzled look, indicating that whomever we were talking to didn't understand. This is the point where we would give up, change the subject into something neutral, and vow to never again try explaining Ray's OCD to anyone (or, if we do talk about it, not to mention his sexual obsessions).

Even though Ray is more open to talking about his OCD, he often hesitates to mention the specifics of his sexual obsessions for many of the same reasons I do. People don't understand. And, he fears what they might think of him because of these obsessions.

ΔΔΔΔ

As of now, most of my friends know that I have OCD. Some of them I have told and there are even a few who have read my first book, ("The Ray of Hope: A Teenager's Fight Against Obsessive Compulsive Disorder"). However, I have never been comfortable openly discussing the specifics of my OCD because of its sexual nature.

Some of my more prying friends have pushed me to talk about my OCD. I can remember sitting with one of my friends at his home, and I told him that I had published a book. He asked, "What kind of book?" Here I was stuck, as I did not want to tell him about my OCD because of the risk the conversation would focus on my particular type of OCD. But, I was obliged to answer. I told him that it was a book that focused on helping people who have OCD. He then asked, "Like where you wash your hands all the time?" I responded "yes," but then, he asked about my OCD. I essentially lied to him about the nature of my OCD. I did not want to be stuck in an awkward conversation if I told him that I was deathly afraid of semen and molesting children. He may have misinterpreted my obsessions and thought of me as a sexual deviant rather than a victim of OCD. I am not, nor will I ever be, comfortable with telling someone about

*the specifics of my OCD (other than those who have OCD, of course).
I worry that if I say too much about my sexual obsessions that others
may wonder if I am dangerous for having such disturbing thoughts.*

*However, even though I worry about what people might
think about my sexual obsessions, I do want to talk more about my
OCD. If I let more people know about my experience then perhaps,
they may be more willing to help those around them who have OCD.
I have told people about my OCD who I think are more understanding, such as a few teachers and some medical professionals. In fact,
one physical therapist I once had for a knee injury even recommended my book to her niece who was suffering from OCD. Gratification
like that keeps me wanting to tell more people about my OCD, but
still I fear being labeled or misinterpreted as a potential criminal.*

ΔΔΔΔ

Why Ray's OCD took on sexual matters as opposed to something else, we have never understood. He could never point to
a certain event in his life and say, "This is where it all started. Because this happened to me, I understand why my OCD focuses on
sexuality." Before understanding all the caveats of OCD, I had worried
that something had happened to Ray. Maybe he had been sexually
abused, and I missed it; maybe he had experimented in sex in an inappropriate way; or maybe he had witnessed someone participating
in a sexually-deviant act. When asked about these ideas, Ray only
remembered one time when he and his friend were surfing the internet and stumbled onto a pornographic site. He says they quickly
exited the site worrying that his friend's parents might come along
and see what they were doing. Exactly what Ray felt during the few
moments when he saw the images on the site, he can't remember. Did he feel sexual excitement, but misinterpret it as something

115

bad? Did his friend say something during that time which confused or embarrassed him? Did he worry that because they were so concerned about hiding their actions from his friend's parents that what they were doing was something to feel guilty about? Ray can't say; he doesn't remember feeling and thinking anything negative during this time. Also, because his sexual obsessions didn't start up until about two years after he and his friend looked at the site, it doesn't make sense that this one instance was what sparked his OCD.

As many parents do when their kid has a mental disorder, I worried that the fault was mine. Maybe I had done something to create Ray's OCD, either in its entirety, or partially, by creating enough steps that allowed it to enter his life. When I searched my own history for any reason that Ray might have sexual obsessions I didn't find much. It was not as if sex was openly discussed in our home; I never dressed in a provocative manner; we didn't have friends who overtly showed their sexuality; and I didn't express disgust or shame regarding sexual topics. And, there was no traumatic event that had ever happened in our family that could be remotely associated with sexuality. There was, however, one minor instance that Ray and I both remember that might have given Ray's OCD an idea to use when it was deciding how to affect Ray.

Our family had recently moved to Shanghai, China because Ray's father had decided to take a sabbatical leave from his university. He took a job teaching, and I found one working as a pediatrician in a Chinese hospital. It was a stressful time, and my mind was busy trying to understand my new home. I was often tired and wanted more time alone so that I could rest, think, and plan. It was during this transition when I decided to no longer sit with Ray during his bath time. Before this, I had always stayed in the bathroom during his bath, spending time with him or talking and reading to him. But one night, I abruptly stopped, mainly for my own selfish reasons. I don't remember exactly what I said, but I remember saying something about him being older (about ten) and that maybe it wasn't appropriate for me to be present during his bath time. Of all the times in my life that I wish it were possible to rewind and listen again to my exact words and see how they were being received, this conversation would top the list. In my memory, Ray didn't react but shrugged and went on to take his bath.

I have often wondered whether my words had somehow triggered in Ray negative feelings about his body. Was it possible that my words caused him to feel shame or guilt about me being present when he was naked, even though he was still a little kid? Did I inadvertently signal to him that what we were doing was wrong and something to be ashamed of? When asked, Ray says he doesn't remember much about this conversation and what he felt afterwards, but he does say one thing that has always stuck with me. He remembers it. If our discussion hadn't had any effect on him, then why does he remember it? Another dilemma regarding the role that this conversation might have had in sparking his OCD is timing. If it had had some negative effect on his thinking, then why did it take over ten months before his OCD latched onto it? Why didn't he start having his sexual obsessions soon after we had talked?

We will never know whether one particular conversation or a pornographic viewing was why Ray's OCD latched onto sexual matters. Perhaps when his OCD was forming, his mind searched for worrisome ideas and readily found the ones regarding sexuality. It's possible that if different emotionally-charged events, such as witnessing violence or being victimized, had been more prominent in his mind, then his OCD wouldn't have taken sexuality as its focus but instead, used violent themes. Maybe OCD is nothing more than an opportunist, taking the easiest path it can find. And for Ray, this path was sexuality.

Many who have OCD are like Ray and have no clue as to why their OCD picks a certain topic. Some, however, can see a connection between their life events and why their OCD took its particular form. Some, for example, can remember a specific event, such as a car wreck, a violent attack, or a life-threatening accident, and draw a direct line from that event to their OCD symptoms. Others can remember a specific comment someone made that triggered their OCD; many times these words are nothing more than off-the-cuff remarks (eg, you parked a little close to that car; you said you would never drive when you had been drinking; you shouldn't have said what you did) but yet, consisted of the right ingredients at the right time to spark an OCD to life. Whether someone who has OCD can pinpoint the reasons for their OCD acting like it does or have no idea, it doesn't matter. I agree with Ray when he says, "If OCD hadn't approached me in the way it did, then it would have appeared in another form." Trying to understand what OCD does or doesn't do, isn't worth the time and effort. It's like trying to understand how tornadoes work while one is bearing down on you. It makes much more sense to figure out how to keep safe.

Ray's sexual obsessions took many forms and were similar to others whose OCD focuses on sexuality. Ray's obsessions, for example, made him incessantly worry that he had hurt someone in a sexual way. For Ray, his thoughts centered mainly on women, both young and old, and how he wasn't sure that he would sexually harm them. He never focused on any individual but worried about all females in general. Others who have sexual obsessions, in contrast, worry about harming a specific person, such as a daughter, a friend of their kids, or a student in their classroom. There are also cases of grandmothers who peer anxiously into their grandchildren's diapers, mothers who are terrified that they will sexually molest their own babies, and fathers who refuse any contact with their daughters because their OCD has convinced them that they can't be trusted. The list of how OCD can hijack sexuality and twist it into something ugly is endless.

Strangely, Ray's sexual obsessions never took on one of the

more common ways in which OCD uses sexuality: He never worried about his sexual orientation. There are many accounts of people with OCD whose main obsessions center on incessantly worrying about whether or not they are homosexual (or heterosexual if they are primarily homosexual). Even though they know that they are sexually attracted to members of the opposite sex, their OCD won't guarantee it. It's like they hear a nonstop mantra in their heads which says things like, "You know you aren't gay, but are you sure you weren't turned on by that man in a tank top that just walked by? How do you know that you aren't a lesbian? Didn't you just look at those woman's breasts and a feel a tingling sensation between your legs?" It's logical that these obsessions could arise because of an old fashioned and unenlightened prejudice against homosexuality, but that's rarely the case. Many who have these obsessions profess no such fear or hatred of those who are homosexual. They just don't feel sure where they are on the sexual spectrum.

One of Ray's rarer, and more fleeting, sexual obsessions centered on nonhumans. On occasion, he would blurt out that he had just looked at one of our cat's bottoms and was worried that he would hurt them in a sexual manner. He had been dealing with his sexual obsessions a long time before this symptom appeared, and it was one of the first to melt away when he started treatment. I never focused on it because it was one of Ray's less boisterous obsessions. Whether others have similar obsessions regarding nonhuman creatures, I'm not sure, but it wouldn't surprise me. Nothing about OCD surprises me anymore. Someone with OCD could walk up to me and tell me that they obsess over having sexual relations with their goldfish, and I wouldn't flinch, laugh out loud, or think anything was wrong with them. I would look them straight in the eye and say something like, "I'm glad you told me about this obsession, now let's see how we can get rid of it."

In the beginning, I worried that the presence of sexual obsessions meant that Ray's OCD would be harder to treat or that he would suffer with it longer than those who obsessed over other things, like dirt and germs. I soon learned, however, that sexual obsessions in OCD are fairly common and are as treatable as other obsessions. One study, which looked at OCD and sexual obsessions, reported that up to 26% of those who have OCD (all adults) who had participated in the study had, at one point, experienced sexual obsessions and that 13% were currently dealing with them. That same study also reported that those who have these obsessions do well in many areas, such as response to treatment, obtaining higher education, getting married, and having families. The only difference this study reported was that those who have sexual obsessions tend to get them earlier in life (about four years) than those who have other types of OCD.

It didn't surprise us to learn that about a quarter of those who have OCD have dealt with sexual obsessions. In fact, my guess for that number would have been higher. I have no way to prove it, but I suspect that a much higher percentage of those who have OCD have had sexual obsessions at one time during their disorder. The reason I think this is based on the conflicts we have regarding sexuality, and in my opinion, this confusion is strong enough to allow OCD a place to grow. OCD is well known for latching onto our greatest fears, and sexuality is one area where many feel uncomfortable. Our sexuality is so personal that most of us never openly talk about it, and we certainly never leave our *Playboys* (or *Playgirls*) sitting on the coffee table for company to see. Also, we're so embarrassed to admit our sexual attractions and preferences that we often resort to humor whenever these topics arise. We can't talk to our kids about sex without feeling anxious, and some of us can't even admit to any personal knowledge on sexual matters. ("No son, your mother and I never had sex. We just found you and your brother in a ditch and brought you home.")

Sex is also routinely indicated as an activity one needs to

fear. When we tell girls to watch out for boys who only want to "get into their pants," we're telling them that there's something dangerous about sexual desires. When boys are chastised for pursuing sexual activities, we're telling them that something is wrong with them or that they are dangerous. Added to this mix is a media that loves to tell us about brutal rapes, sexual abuse, and who's buying the services of prostitutes. With this constant negativity surrounding sex, it makes sense that OCD would readily latch onto it.

Sex is something we desire; we have evolved to participate in it and find it pleasurable, but yet, we are constantly told that sex is sometimes bad. Most of us can navigate our lives confidently knowing whether or not our sexual behavior is acceptable. But for those whose brains are susceptible to OCD, dealing with sexuality can become a problem. Some with OCD can no longer feel assured that their thoughts and actions are appropriate and good. Simply looking at a beautiful woman or a handsome man, for example, can set off a barrage of thoughts in someone who has OCD. "Oh my god, I just looked at that woman's breasts that must mean I want to rape her, or I just felt a sensation in my genital area when I looked at that child, does that mean I'm really a pedophile?" We are also bombarded every day with sexual stimuli; we are reminded of our sexuality almost every waking minute; and we possess internal sensors that are constantly sending us messages about our sexual desires. With all this sexual traffic coming and going, it's a small wonder that more of us don't have negative sexual obsessions.

Ray also has never figured out why his OCD took sexuality as its main topic when he was younger and like me, has decided that it's not worth worrying about.

ΔΔΔΔ

During my worst struggles with OCD, I often wished that my OCD had taken on a topic other than sexuality. I felt that having sexuality as a focus for my OCD was one of the worst possible kinds because of the stigma and embarrassment that surrounds sexual topics. Why my OCD chose this particular topic is also something that I have never understood, and I have wasted countless hours trying to find some clue as to why my OCD took on a sexual nature.

Many of my thoughts revolved around the idea that because I had had a sexual thought, I was a horrible person. My OCD had even gone so far as to make me terrified of the possibility that I had drugged someone and had sexually assaulted them. I remember one time when I was eleven years old and had just returned from a Fourth of July celebration. Shortly after returning home, my OCD started in, and I started obsessing over the possibility that I had hurt someone in a sexual manner. No one, not even my mom, could convince me that I had not actually done something terrible.

Many times, I have wished that I had some other kind of obsession other than sexuality. During the times when I was undergoing therapy for my sexual obsessions, I had also wondered if other types of OCD would have been easier to target with therapy. I don't know about this, but I do know that it would have been much easier to talk to my mom about others topics, such as fearing germs or worrying about door locks, than it was about sex.

Where do I think my sexual obsessions came from? I honestly no longer worry about this. I am sure that if my obsessions had not been sexual in nature, my OCD would have picked another topic.   When I think about my past, I cannot find anything that would have triggered my sexual obsessions. I never experienced any type of shock or abuse that would make me respond negatively or be more sensitive to sexuality. My only guess as to why my OCD took on its sexual nature is the current societal view towards sexuality and towards sexual offenses in particular.

When we look at those who have been imprisoned, we often think of prisoners who have sexually preyed on children as the most evil. Our society considers sexual predators as the most deplorable people on the planet, and many times, we see this idea portrayed in our media. Thus, it does not seem unusual that OCD would strike upon such a gold mine of anxiety-provoking thoughts. No one of decency and respectability would ever think of hurting someone in a sexual manner, so it's not surprising that OCD would latch onto this topic. After all, OCD often targets that which we fear the most.

ΔΔΔΔ

Because sexual (and violent) obsessions could easily be misinterpreted, I suggest to anyone who has these obsessions to be cautious when talking about their OCD. I don't say this because these obsessions are shameful but because the world is full of people who say and act without understanding the specifics of many situations (think talk radio). I would hate for anyone who has sexual obsessions to figuratively end up in the same pile as sex offenders. It would only take a few loud mouths with short attention spans and overactive imaginations to ruin someone's standing in the community or maybe even cause the loss of friends, jobs, and opportunities. I think it's much safer for anyone who has sexual obsessions to talk mainly with us, their fellow sufferers of OCD, with their mental health professionals, or with trusted family and friends.

Finally, I would like to personally address those with OCD who have sexual obsessions. Even though you may feel low, despicable, and unworthy because of your obsessions, I trust you. Many of you worry that you would hurt others, especially little kids, but I know different. In fact, I would trust you with little children more than anyone else. And, I am one who has learned the hard way not to easily trust. As a pediatrician, I have been fooled by many who have abused, neglected, and hurt kids. Seemingly upstanding citizens, who had frequented my office, were later identified as rapists and abusers. Because of these experiences, I learned to look harder at those around me and to suspect problems at the smallest hint. But, I know you are not among these child molesters. I would have no concerns placing you in a room with small children and walking away. You would never hurt them; your OCD makes you ever so vigilant to your words and actions that in a strange way, it makes you more trustworthy, not less. Weird, isn't it? But, I also need to remind you that you don't need to keep your OCD around to maintain my trust.

Part III – Treatment With Exposure and Response Prevention Therapy (ERP)

Introduction to ERP

When Ray first started his exposure and response prevention (ERP) therapy, he had too many OCD symptoms to count, but by the time he had trudged through three large ERP sessions and one small one, his OCD was almost invisible. The process had been incredible to witness, almost like watching someone who was initially paralyzed, progress from taking small and tentative steps to running a marathon. This process, however, had not been a linear and predictable one, but instead, was winding and confusing. Some parts of his therapy that I thought would surely propel Ray forward failed, whereas others pleasantly surprised us by their effect. There were also times when Ray's OCD improved amazingly fast, and I thought he would reach his goals within a short time, but then suddenly, we found ourselves plodding uncertainly along, like we had ran out of road and had been forced to blaze a new trail. What I would tell anyone who is attempting to take this journey is to be prepared for anything, expect setbacks but don't be surprised by them, and to take heart by every step forward.

Before Ray's ERP sessions, I didn't dare to dream that OCD could really be controlled and that he could have an OCD-free life. I had accepted the idea that OCD would always be in charge, telling Ray what he could do, where he could go, and who he could talk to. I had envisioned Ray's future where he had to consult the ever-present OCD before any decision could be made. These are the thoughts I had before we learned about and then implemented ERP.

If there is one word to describe the effects of ERP, it would be this: Magic. When I watched Ray's OCD break after his first ERP session it was like the magic spell had been found that was powerful enough to cast OCD out. Never before in my life had I seen anything so dramatic and impressive. Where OCD once looked impenetrable, it was now crumbling around our feet. For us, it was like we had brought down a mountain that had been standing in our way and was one that we never dreamed could be moved.

Even though ERP works magic when appropriately applied, it's not a cure for OCD. OCD is not a condition that can be completely eliminated; it will always lurk in those who have it. But with ERP, a cage can be built that is strong enough to hold whatever form OCD tries to take. Any monster that's confined to its cage is powerless. My advice to anyone who continues to struggle with OCD is this: Use ERP to build a strong cage, coax OCD into it, slam the door shut, and never look back. And please, never, ever, feed the damn thing.

Describing ERP

The main treatment for OCD is exposure and response prevention therapy (ERP). The description of ERP is deceptively simple: Face your fears (ie, your obsessions), don't perform your compulsions that you normally do in response to your obsessions, and in time, the obsessions will go away. If, for example, someone obsessively thinks that their hands are dirty and because of these thoughts, they compulsively wash their hands, then for their ERP, they would be expected to touch something unclean (eg, a garbage can) and not wash their hands. Even though they would feel extreme anxiety in the beginning of this exercise, they would soon start to feel that anxiety decrease. This happens because our bodies can't maintain high levels of anxiety for long times. (The official term for what happens during ERP is habituation.) One way to understand this is to remember how in a new environment certain sounds are annoying at first, but in time, those same sounds fade into the background. This is what happens during ERP; in time and with continued exposure, obsessions fade away. They no longer register as something important, and without any attention to feed them, obsessions turn into just thoughts.

The main problem with doing ERP is simple to understand. ERP is frightening. To those whose obsessions feel real, asking them to face down those obsessions without any help (ie, doing their compulsions) is like asking them to jump out of an airplane without a parachute. Trying to describe what ERP feels like and why it causes so much fear isn't easy. One analogy that I have tried using is as follows: Doing ERP is like asking someone to jump into what they see as a raging fire. Those of us who are supporting them tell them that the fire isn't real and that they need to trust us when we say that they will be fine after they jump. They also need to make this jump even though all their senses tell them differently. What appears before them sounds, smells, looks, and feels like a real fire. They put their hands up to it, and it feels hot; in fact, they can even feel the pain that a real fire would cause. "You are crazy if you want me to jump into this fire," they scream. "You must hate me if you expect me to do this. It will kill me. Are you sure there is no other way?" Only after a lot of explaining, cajoling, begging, pleading, and maybe even bribing, are they convinced to jump. But, it's not done. Because when they jump, what do they immediately feel? Not relief, but a searing pain that threatens to completely unnerve them. All their instincts tell them to jump back out of the fire to their perceived safety. But, if they can be convinced to take the pain for just a few seconds, something amazing happens. They realize that the fire (ie, their obsessions) wasn't real and that their pain is dwindling faster than they ever could have imagined. Soon, the fire starts to die and within a short time, it's gone. "Can it really be," they ask in wonderment, "that the fire was never real to begin with? How could I have been fooled all that time into believing that it was real?" They then understand that even though their fire appeared real to them, no else could feel it. But for ERP to really work, one jump into the fire isn't good enough. Successful ERP requires repeated jumping over a short time period and will probably also require the jumping into new fires (ie, new obsessions) that have been started. Overcoming the fear the first time, however, makes it easier. Anyone who has survived the first jump into the fire understands that the pain they initially feel will quickly fade. With persistent ERP, someone with OCD can reach the point when all the burning fires that had raged around them are reduced to nothing more than small, smoldering embers.

Here's Ray's description of ERP and what he felt while undergoing it.

ΔΔΔΔ

When asked to describe ERP, I often try to evoke a metaphor that captures the complex nature of ERP therapy and its impact on the person with OCD. ERP is difficult and terrifying at the time of action, but as the therapy becomes more effective, both the difficulty and fear turn out to be embarrassing in retrospect. Even today, I still marvel at the lengths I took to avoid a bathroom in my house that I feared was contaminated or the hours I put into washing my hands each week. Only through ERP did I realize that all of my obsessions and compulsions were ridiculous. But at the time when I started therapy, I had no idea that this was the realization that ERP would allow me to have.

There is a film called "The Village" that perfectly encapsulates the way ERP makes you feel as well as the realizations that ERP brings. In this film, there is a village run by a group of elders who, through fear, persuade all of the village inhabitants that in the forest that surrounds the border of their village dwell creatures that will kill anyone who attempts to enter the forest. The elders even go so far as to make costumes and to pretend that they are the dreaded creatures, making sure that they are sighted on occasion. Because of this, the people in the village are terrified of the forest and live their whole lives thinking that any attempt to leave the village will result in death. Due to this fear, the villagers do not have access to technology like the rest of the modern world and many have to suffer through illnesses that are easily treatable, despite the fact that their elders know that they can get medicine from outside the village. Eventually, one villager decides to leave the village and enter the forest to seek help for a sick loved one. She feels intense fear during the travel through the forest due to her lifelong fear of the forest until she finally makes it through and really understands that the elders made up the fear to keep all of the villagers from leaving. Not only did she feel relieved after learning the truth about the forest, but she also felt angry and embarrassed for living her whole life under an irrational fear.

This is precisely the way ERP made me feel both at the beginning and the end of my therapy. When confronted with the idea of facing something like touching my pants and not washing my hands, I remember feeling anxiety bubble uncontrollably, resulting in an anger and fear that I could not control. Also, even after I was motivated enough to go through the ERP, I was terrified during the process and remained in shambles afterwards. But then, I eventually felt a realization pass over me that nothing had gone wrong and that maybe my fear was based on nothing but the whims of a bully like OCD (much like the elders in "The Village"). After surviving several ERP sessions, I actually felt embarrassed over how long I had been scared of such trivial things such as walking into a bathroom in my house or petting one of my cats.

Another metaphor that describes ERP and its effects is the fear of public speaking. Many people hate public speaking and often rank it as one of the things most feared besides death. However, the fear of speaking in public is irrational when one thinks about it. What harm really comes out of it if one fails to do it well? There is no physical harm that can come from addressing a crowd, and the most that can happen is a little embarrassment if the speech goes horribly. And, one can always practice their speech to ensure that it goes well. Also, after a speech is given, the most common feeling felt is the realization of the absurdity of fearing public speaking. I remember when I had to give a forty-five minute keynote address about my first book to a crowd of around 150 people. The fear I felt prior to the speech was so great that I regretted that I had ever agreed to give the speech. Once I gave the speech, however, I smacked my head in embarrassment at the hours of wasted thought that I had devoted to worrying about that speech. Giving the speech was a lot like doing ERP. Once it was done, I was amazed as to how good I felt.

Motivation to do ERP

Telling someone who has OCD that the treatment they need to undertake (ie, ERP) is complicated, time consuming, and frightening practically guarantees that they won't want to hear any more about it. In an era where there is a pill or procedure for most medical ailments, ERP seems too primitive, like applying leeches or performing demon exorcisms. How is a loved one or therapist to motivate someone who has OCD to undertake ERP when it seems so difficult and uncertain?

For some with OCD, the motivation is already in place. Someone who is older and has long-standing OCD has already experienced its many negative effects such as job losses, divorces, family discord, and other health issues. These people know what devastation OCD can cause and are ready to face it. They may have even hit bottom and have nowhere to go but up. In other words, OCD has already taken everything away, and they have nothing left to lose. For these folks, ERP doesn't seem so bad.

In a cable program that showed patients with OCD and their therapists using ERP (A&E's *Obsessed*), it was evident that most had become motivated to fight their OCD because they had experienced a lot of loss because of it. Some had lost jobs and were too engrossed in their OCD to look for new ones. Many saw how their OCD was negatively affecting their children and wanted to rid themselves of their OCD so that they could parent better. Others wanted to attend college but couldn't because their compulsions took up so much of their time. All these reasons are good ones for wanting to get better, but when I watched these programs I wondered: Is it possible to motivate someone to do ERP before so much loss has occurred? How far would Ray have to fall before I could convince him to try ERP?

It is also hard to understand why someone who has OCD and is suffering from it won't try the very treatment that can alleviate that suffering. One barrier to treatment that was present for Ray was that his compulsions were comforting. He felt better after he washed his hands or after he confessed his bad thoughts. This is why compulsions are so powerful; they help alleviate the anxiety caused by the obsessions. I know that Ray often wanted me to stay out of his way and let him do his compulsion because performing these compulsions were his only source of comfort. But as anyone who routinely deals with OCD knows, any comfort that is provided by a compulsion is fleeting, and the need to redo yet another compulsion comes up quickly, sometimes only within seconds after completing the first one. Ray also experienced an escalating need to perform his compulsions. Where one hand washing per hour used to work, it became ten or even twenty. Where one confession per hour used to suffice, it became too many to count. At his worst, Ray would do anything to get that temporary feeling of relief, not unlike a druggie looking for his next hit.

By the time we were considering ERP, Ray OCD's had been active for over a year. He was on medication and had tried talk therapy, both professionally and with me, but his OCD showed no signs of waning. Many cognitive maneuvers had been tried in an attempt to dislodge OCD from his brain. It had repeatedly been pointed out to him, for example, that his obsessions were irrational, how just because someone has certain thoughts it doesn't mean that they will ever act on those thoughts, how everyone has similar types of thoughts as his obsessions but find ways to let these thoughts go by, and how if he would give less meaning to his obsessions that they would go away. But even with all this explaining, his life was still miserable and under OCD's control. Most of his thoughts were still OCD related and most of his actions were centered on alleviating the anxiety caused by OCD.

All the pain and misery that OCD was causing Ray still wasn't strong enough for him to seriously consider ERP. Even after it was explained to him that ERP was the treatment OCD experts used on their patients and that it had been proven effective for treating OCD, he still didn't want anything to do with it. OCD was causing him great pain and loss, but he wasn't yet motivated to try ERP. At this point, I wondered how much more pain would he endure and how much more he would lose before he would try ERP. And, how much more time would go by? Would it take another year or would it be ten years of living with OCD before he decided to actively work on it? Was it possible that he would resort to drugs or alcohol as a way to deal with his intense anxiety or even contemplate suicide before he considered ERP a viable option? I was also unsure about my own role. Was it reasonable for me to stand back and let him fall? Maybe I should go on with my own life and wait until he was ready to try harder. Or, could I find another way? Could motivation to do ERP come from a source other than one's desire to live without OCD? In other words, was it possible to shift motivation to do ERP from an intrinsic source to an extrinsic one?

Even though he couldn't explain it at the time when his OCD was the most active, Ray can now offer some ideas as to why he was initially so resistant to doing ERP.

ΔΔΔΔ

Mustering the courage to do ERP was undoubtedly the biggest roadblock for me in getting over OCD. Strangely, I knew that I had a problem with my OCD; I even had the tools and knowledge to overcome it, yet the fear of doing the therapy prevented me from implementing them. Despite having done hours of cognitive reasoning into the absurdity of my OCD thoughts and listening to my mom explain to me about how ERP would help me, I was always at square one when asked to do ERP. I also had a large quantity of petrifying fear when it came to confronting my OCD thoughts. So here was my biggest problem: How do I obtain the motivation and drive not only to start doing ERP but to follow it through to the end?

OCD is relentless in attacking one's morality. Every day my OCD convinced me that because of something I did, I hurt someone else. This resulted in me believing that I was an evil person. I cannot count the number of times I thought that I was one of the most evil persons in the world. Because of this twisted thinking, I tried hard to avoid anything that would trigger my obsessions. But with ERP, you actually have to perform the very actions that trigger your OCD thoughts, and to me, it was like I was being asked to perform something evil. Even though I tried using logic, I was still not convinced that by performing the actions that triggered my obsessions, I could get better. I continued to believe that my compulsions kept the world safe from me, an evil person.

My mom understood that for me to get better, we had to do ERP. At first, she tried to convince me that OCD was ruining my life and that to get rid of OCD I had to do ERP. This type of rhetoric proved useless as I was still convinced that my actions were protecting people. By washing my hands after accidently touching my pants or confessing every questionable thought I had, I believed that I was preventing the moral desecration of someone. In other words, I was too scared to give up my compulsions.

There was a small part of me, however, that knew my obsessions were not real and that my compulsions did nothing but keep me enslaved. I think this part stayed alive by the repeated efforts of my mom; she told me every day that my obsessions were not based on reality and that once I accepted that idea, I could get better. It was to this part of me that she made an appeal for trying ERP. But she also knew that more talking wouldn't help me overcome my fears; it would require something stronger, much stronger.

What my mom did was to make me an offer I couldn't refuse. She would pay me, and pay me well, to do ERP.

ΔΔΔΔ

Once I finally understood that Ray wouldn't readily give up his compulsions because he believed that they were keeping the world safe from his "evil" thoughts, I realized that a different approach would be needed. Since appealing to his logical mind had failed, I decided to try accessing a different area of his brain. I hoped that we could use it to override Ray's faulty OCD circuits and convince him to give up his compulsions. The brain area (or pathway) that we used was one that all people use every day of their lives: The reward pathway. And, we would access Ray's reward pathway by using money.

Within the last few decades, neuroscientists have located, mapped, and defined many different areas of the brain. Many of these areas are now known to be specialized and perform certain activities, such as processing sensory information (ie, hearing, sight, and touch), performing motor activities, processing emotion, and executing plans. One area that has been extensively studied is called the reward pathway. This pathway, which also exists in animals, is important for our survival because it helps us to seek out pleasurable experiences, such as eating food or having sex. Without this pathway, it's possible that our species wouldn't have survived because our ancestors might not have eaten enough or sought out mates to have children. Scientists have also found that in addition to eating and procreating, we use our reward pathway to experience and enjoy a wide range of experiences. Whenever we experience something that feels good, such as helping someone, solving a problem, acquiring money, or even donating to a charity, we are using the reward pathway. We like to feel good, and we seek out those experiences that allow us to access that good feeling. And, we do this many times a day, every day of our lives. In other words, our reward pathways are like superhighways, well traveled, easily accessible, and well connected.

I knew it was the right decision to pay Ray to do ERP the second I made my offer. I could almost see his reward pathway firing up and coming on line. Where before all I saw was fear and uncertainty about ERP, I now saw hope and possibility. Instead of focusing on all that could go wrong during ERP, Ray was thinking about what he could buy with his money. I now had hope that at least, Ray would approach ERP and give it a real try.

Many therapists and parents would probably disagree with the idea of paying a teenager to undergo ERP. When I first described this idea to others, I was often met with skepticism and was even discouraged from following through with it. On one level their arguments made sense. Shouldn't Ray do ERP because it was the right way to treat his OCD? Wouldn't it be best for him in the long run to understand that ERP was necessary and that he should do it because it was good for him, like doing his homework or brushing his teeth? We don't pay our kids to do many things in their lives that are important to them, such as going to school or following the rules we teach them. So, why should ERP be different? What I often said to those who questioned my idea of paying Ray to do ERP was that all of their ideas had been tried and had failed. OCD was unlike anything that most of them had ever faced. It isn't a simple discipline problem that responds to punishment; it isn't an issue that can be talked through to a solution; and it certainly isn't a phase that can be weathered through. The usual rules of parenting don't apply to OCD and its therapy.

One worry that I had with regards to paying Ray to do ERP was its long-term effect. Would he think less of me for resorting to bribery instead of taking a higher, more moralistic road? Would he always need a substantial reward to fight off his OCD or would he learn to take care of it on his own? What would happen to his OCD when he got older and no longer lived at home where I could provide the necessary reinforcements? Ray can now answer these questions.

ΔΔΔΔ

After much deliberation, we found that money was the motivating factor to get me through ERP. With the money in mind, I could momentarily ignore my OCD thoughts that were screaming at me to wash my hands, change my clothes, or confess my thoughts. I was also able to override most of my anxiety by thinking of what I could acquire with my money. In a sense, my well-established, yet false, morality that had been imposed by OCD was being corrupted by the allure of cash. It worked like a charm.

After we discovered how powerful money was in motivating me to fight my OCD, what we needed most then was time and patience to see what ERP could do. I cannot stress how important rewards are when undergoing ERP therapy. After all, doing ERP is painful and without any tangible reward, there is little motivation to do it. It would be like working in a coal mine all day without pay. As of now, I no longer need any type of extrinsic reward or incentive to fight my OCD because I now know how much better life is without OCD. On the occasion when my OCD springs up, I am able to fight it back using the tools I learned.

Understandably, the rewards granted for doing ERP will vary from person to person. After all, an adult cannot rely on their parents for cash rewards nor can all parents provide cash rewards to their children. However, it is vital that some kind of reward system be discovered and implemented if OCD is to be defeated. Adults could perhaps use improved family relationships or better job opportunities as incentives to undergo ERP. Young children might be convinced for as little as ice cream or a trip to the zoo. Teenagers, however, might prove more difficult. Even if money is not readily available, other incentives, such as staying out later with friends, having their own room at home, or more time with the family car, might work.

ΔΔΔΔ

Even though using money as an incentive to work on ERP proved effective for us, there were many nuances involved in its actual application. In fact, there was a lot of trial and error before we found the right formula. Initially, I had tried tying a weekly allowance into a set of chore-like activities that involved OCD. Ray would be given, for example, $20 if he accomplished certain exposures, such as touching a particular doorknob five times during the week, restricting his hand washing to three times each evening, using only five squirts of hand soap for each hand washing, and restricting his showering to one time each day. One problem with this approach was that it took a lot of vigilance on my part. I had to keep score and to watch Ray constantly to make sure he didn't cheat by seeking in an extra hand washing or using extra soap when I wasn't watching. I also had to constantly patrol the kitchen and bathroom areas like a cop on the beat. The other problem with this approach was that the exposures we used were too small to make a difference. Because Ray was in school and the main time we had was in the evenings, there weren't many hours (or spare mental energy) to spend in attempting larger and more difficult exposures. As a result, Ray's OCD only minimally improved using this small cash for small exposures approach.

Another idea I tried was to use a large sum of money to entice Ray to expose himself to something large and scary. Instead of starting small and working our way up to the more hairy exposures, we would try tackling one of his worst fears. For a long time, Ray had refused to even step into a certain bathroom in our home. His OCD had convinced him that this bathroom was especially contaminated with sexual material, and because of these thoughts, Ray feared this room more than any other. He even tried to keep everyone else from using this bathroom and would repeatedly ask me who had used it. His fear of this area was so intense that at one time, we dubbed it the "evil bathroom." Because of his intense fear, I thought that if he could face this bathroom, then maybe his OCD would quickly back down. With this in mind, I offered him several hundred dollars to stand in that bathroom for several minutes. I chose such a large sum because I knew that he was being asked to do something that, in his mind, was like being asked to undergo surgery without anesthesia. After thinking about it, he decided to try. The end result was that he stood in the bathroom for several minutes, took his money, ran with it, and then refused to even talk about the bathroom for several months.

What finally worked was to promise Ray a moderate sum, like a salary, to work on his OCD over a defined time period, such as one to two weeks. It was also important that during this time, OCD was the primary focus and not school, friends, or hanging out. It became like a focused business project that required completion before payment was delivered. By the end of his ERP therapy, Ray had been paid to complete several of these "projects," and I was amazed by the results. When we had finished, Ray had markedly improved, and his OCD was no longer the primary force in his life. The payoff from my investments was worth every penny and more.

My experience with paying Ray to do ERP was a little like *Goldilocks and the Three Bears*. We had tried too little and too much before we found what was just right. I don't know if what worked for Ray will also work for others who have OCD. But, I do know that if it hadn't been for the money, I don't know how else we could have started, let alone continued, ERP.

Finding Help For ERP

Where else in the medical arena does the following situation exist? There is a well-established and proven treatment for a condition, but many who have that condition fail either to receive the treatment or if they do, fail to receive an adequate version of that treatment. This is what often happens in OCD. When those of us with OCD ask for help from mental health professionals, we are often not provided with the treatment that is considered the standard of care. Anywhere else in medicine, this failure would result in those professionals being sanctioned or removed from their positions. I have often wondered how much quicker those who have OCD could improve their symptoms if mental health professionals were held accountable to the same degree as other medical professionals.

Even though ERP is the treatment that experts cite as the most effective for OCD, not all mental health professional who treat OCD use ERP. There are even some who haven't heard of it or dismiss it as an intervention they don't believe actually works. Why so many in the mental health profession fail to adequately use ERP for the treatment of OCD has never been clear to me. Is it that ERP is too new and not enough time has passed for it to become part of the necessary curriculums? Maybe not enough studies have been done to convince all those, who are involved in treating OCD, to change their methods. Or, maybe the professions responsible for treating OCD are not ones that insist on keeping up to date on the latest methods. It is also possible that implementing ERP is too difficult for many professionals to master and that specialists, who are specifically trained to use ERP, are necessary. If ERP is ever to be routinely used for the treatment of OCD, it's necessary for all these barriers to be indentified and torn down.

How many in the mental health profession fail to use ERP for treating OCD is not clear. Perhaps it's only a small proportion, and it's my thinking on this that's wrong. Sadly, I don't think so. Even though I haven't found studies that directly address the number of mental health professionals who fail to use ERP for treating OCD, I did find information that suggests that the sufferers of other psychiatric maladies are also not receiving the care they should. One article that I found cited research that stated that psychiatric patients in the U.S. and Britain rarely receive cognitive behavioral therapy (CBT) even though scientific research has proven that this therapy is effective for conditions like depression and anxiety. This article also stated that of 200 psychologists, only 17% of them used exposure therapy (ERP is a form of CBT) with patients who have post-traumatic stress disorder (a type of anxiety disorder where someone remains anxious after experiencing a traumatic event) even though scientific studies have proven that it's effective for these patients. Also, of those patients who have eating disorders, it has been reported that fewer than half of them have received the treatment that has been proven effective for their disorder. The reasons for why mental health professionals fail to use the interventions that have been scientifically proven to help are not clear. One idea is that perhaps too many therapists view their work as more like art rather than science and because of this, fail to look at the scientific literature when deciding how to treat their patients.

With the continued efforts of professional organizations, such as the International OCD Foundation and the Anxiety and Depression Association of America, I hope that ERP will eventually reach into all corners of the mental health profession and that ERP will become as standard a treatment to OCD as chemotherapy is to cancer. Also, as more of us who have OCD regain our mental health through ERP and tell our stories to those who are still struggling, we will force the mental health professionals to pay attention. What better way is there to force changes other than success?

Unfortunately for Ray, the mental health professional we

first went to didn't use ERP to address Ray's OCD. Instead he used talk therapy, which has been proven ineffective for OCD.

ΔΔΔΔ

When my mom and I finally accepted that my actions and thoughts were a result of OCD and that we needed help, we went to and dutifully returned to a psychologist, who in retrospect, had minimal experience with OCD. Out of convenience, location, and cost, we decided that he was the best option we had. As it turned out, this psychologist was neither insightful to my OCD or all that friendly, so I was intimidated by him and did not come close to confiding in him the nature of my OCD. After describing my thoughts to him, he tried pushing me into thinking that to overcome my thoughts, I would have to think about them in a completely different way and utilize my human gift of logic to convince myself that they did not make sense. One particular example of this was when I told my psychologist that I had an immense fear of a certain bathroom in our home because I thought it was contaminated with sexual material. He spent the entire hour of our session trying to persuade me of and then guide me through the deductions as to why that notion of a contaminated bathroom was absurd. At the end of the session, he told tell me that when I got home, I needed to go into that bathroom. This never worked because I was too scared and didn't have anyone pushing or guiding me. After about two months of visiting this psychologist, my OCD wasn't much better, and we were frustrated with hours of wasted time and wasted money. At this point, my mom and I were convinced that this psychologist was not going to help us.

ΔΔΔΔ

Deciding to use ERP as a treatment for OCD was only the first step in a long and winding path to actually executing an ERP plan. As the saying goes, "The devil is in the details." And, ERP requires the handling of endless details. One of the first and important steps to take is to decide who is responsible for making and then implementing the ERP plan. Ideally, this person should be a mental health professional (eg, psychologist, psychiatrist, or social worker) who has received training in ERP. Such trained professionals, however, are not easy to find, especially in more rural areas. As for us, our previous and negative experiences in dealing with the mental health community left us hesitant to try again. This left us with few choices. We could dig harder and try finding a local therapist who uses ERP, try to locate one who was farther away and spend hours driving, or attempt ERP ourselves.

Whenever one is faced with something as complicated as OCD, the most reasonable step to take is to look high and low for the right therapist, turn over every rock, follow every lead, and don't stop until the most qualified and dedicated person is found. Finding such a person, however, is only the first step because inevitably, they will be booked for months on end. Good therapists for OCD are hard to find, and they will always have more work than what they can possibly handle. I wonder what I would have done if I had found an ERP therapist close by but was told that they weren't accepting any new patients. Most likely, I would have resorted to begging, crying, pleading, and maybe even, lying; I would have done whatever it took to get my son to that therapist.

Unfortunately, hiring a therapist is also a situation of "buyer beware." There are many therapists who claim expertise in treating OCD, but who don't use ERP. Many will state outright that they have successfully treated people who have OCD and that they are comfortable handling even the worst cases. But, these reassurances are far from adequate. Anyone who needs help with their OCD should dig deep and be prepared to ask many questions. Ideally, during a therapist interview one (or a parent) should hear some version of the following: "I have successfully used exposure and response prevention therapy to treat 100's of people (kids) who have OCD. I have seen and have helped those who have different types of OCD, such contamination fears, intrusive thoughts, including violent and sexual obsessions, and symmetry or "just right" obsessions. I am comfortable using different techniques in ERP, such as having my patients use real exposures or having them use mental imagery. I am willing to push you (your child) into doing exposures but will never be abusive nor will I ever use shame. I am also willing to travel to your home or wherever it's necessary because often, the most effective exposures need to be done in environments outside of my office." If I had ever heard a therapist say these things, I would have dropped to the floor and kissed their feet. I might even have offered them all my worldly goods if they had added, "I have also attended the Behavior Therapy Training Institute that is offered by the International OCD Foundation, and I attend the annual OCD conference every year so that I can learn even more about how to treat OCD."

In our rural area, searching for a good OCD therapist is like trying to find the proverbial needle in a haystack. I considered trying to find a haystack that had more needles in it, that is, widening our search to include more urban areas. But, I quickly lost heart. Even if we did find an OCD therapist in our closest city, it would mean hours of traveling and a lot of missed school for Ray. And, what if Ray didn't connect well with a new therapist even though they were well trained in handling OCD? We easily could end up wasting a lot of time, money, and effort and still not have dented Ray's OCD. What were we to do then? Try yet another therapist and spend even more time and money in the hopes of finding the one who would save us?

Another option I briefly considered was having Ray admitted to an inpatient facility that specializes in treating OCD or an extensive outpatient program where he would attend an OCD treatment facility for several hours each day for several weeks. Scattered throughout the U.S. are several OCD treatment facilities that have programs which are specifically designed to use ERP therapy and are staffed by experts who know how to implement the therapy (a list of these programs is located on the International OCD Foundation website). Maybe if Ray had continued his downward spiral and had become so dysfunctional that he couldn't attend school or leave the house, I would have pursued this option further. But, Ray wasn't there yet, and I felt that we still had other ideas to try first.

With no good therapist close by and with no heart to travel far to find one, we opted to take a third and unusual path: I would be Ray's new therapist, and we would try ERP on our own. It was mostly out of desperation, mixed with a little lunacy, that this decision was reached. It was not out of arrogance or disdain. It was more like a Hail Mary pass that was being made by players who were out of good ideas. And, there was the fear. Ray's OCD had been in control of his life for a long time, and I feared that it would never let go. How much more could he take before he gave up ever having a normal and healthy life? Maybe we could have safely waited for several more months to see what would happen with a new therapist or to see if the OCD would somehow magically lessen, but I was too scared to take that chance. Each day that OCD was in charge of Ray's mind was a day that was lost to him. Sometimes, I swear I could even sense his brain tearing itself apart trying to fight off the OCD. How many more neurons would be sacrificed in this seemingly endless battle? It was time to start fighting back, and if I had to lead the charge, then so be it.

When I made the decision to direct Ray's therapy I knew that it was a crazy thing to consider trying. We were desperate and were having a difficult time finding help, but could I really help Ray do ERP?

I knew that I didn't have the qualifications to undertake my son's therapy. I loved him and wanted the best for him, but was I really capable of directing his therapy and was it even possible that I could do more harm than good? I didn't know when we started ERP what would happen, but at the time, I decided that it was worth a try and forged ahead. It was only after we had started our ERP sessions that I came across this sentence in an OCD book, "Several studies have found that exposure therapy can be just as effective when it is self-administered as when a therapist is involved." The same paragraph also mentioned that someone might want to find a trusted friend or family member to help if they find that they can't do it on their own. Not surprisingly, it was also said that if someone's problem is severe that they should consult a qualified mental health professional. After reading this, I realized that maybe what we were attempting wasn't so crazy after all and that our chance of success was higher than what I had originally hoped.

Getting Started With ERP

Even after we had acquired our weapon (ie, ERP) to use for fighting OCD and had decided on a leader (ie, me), we still had to solve several problems. One of the obvious ones was that we had to find an appropriate date and time to implement our ERP plan. And, we had to decide how much time was needed. Would a series of small bites do or should we take huge chunks at one time? Was it possible to take an hour out of a day, such as after school, evenings, or on weekends, and make real progress on OCD? Or, was doing ERP more like trying to push a large rock up a hill, a situation where smaller efforts amount to nothing and only results in exhaustion? Maybe doing ERP requires large, coordinated efforts that are made over a short time period, just like the ones that are needed to move a large rock.

Ray and I had tried doing ERP on a mini scale, hoping that the smaller, less painful steps would suffice and that we wouldn't have to dedicate large amounts of time for ERP. It didn't work; it was like trying to put out a large fire with a squirt gun. We then had to find the chunks of time where Ray and I could stop our lives and focus on doing ERP. Since I was no longer working outside the home, I could drop any previous plans I had and take up working on ERP, but for Ray it wasn't as easy. He was in high school and knew that taking time away from his studies was a huge risk to his future. Gaps in one's academic record always stand out and explaining those holes is often problematic. And even if we tried taking a few, intermittent days by calling him in sick, there was always the worry that the stress and effort of doing ERP would render him exhausted and ineffective when he did return to school.

Since after school and during school wasn't feasible for working on ERP, our only remaining choices were the times between school sessions. That is, could we use school breaks, such as Christmas, spring, and summer breaks, for ERP? Needless to say,

Ray wasn't thrilled with this idea but eventually realized that these times were the best suited for our purposes. These breaks were long enough for intensive sessions on ERP and were positioned so that Ray's grades wouldn't be affected. It meant, of course, that Ray would have to give up his downtime to work on ERP. It was like being asked to work on a difficult, dirty, and nasty project during one's vacation instead of traveling to someplace fun and exciting.

Overall, Ray also felt that his vacation time was a good time to work on ERP.

ΔΔΔΔ

During my worst periods of OCD, I never wanted to travel or go on any sort of vacation because I was too afraid of situations that would put me under too much anxiety. I did not want to stay at a hotel because I knew that I would have to share a bathroom with others, a situation that was sure to trigger my OCD. If that happened, then I knew that my worries would consume all of my waking thoughts and that I would be forced to endure pure anxiety until I found a place where I could perform my compulsions of hand washing.

Giving up my vacation time to do ERP therapy was actually not as hard as some may think. Because we stayed home most of the time during my school vacations, I had plenty of time to do ERP exposures. Also, because my mom had offered me a cash reward for doing these exposures I could think of ERP as more like work that had to be done if I wanted my rewards. If it hadn't been for the rewards, however, I probably would have thought differently about giving up my vacations to do ERP.

ΔΔΔΔ

One of the challenging parts to doing ERP is deciding on the actual steps to take. Most OCD books that are written by professionals approach this by advising the development of an exposure hierarchy as a first step. In principle, what this consists of is simple: Make a list of the triggers for one's obsessions starting with the least anxiety provoking and then working the way up to the most frightening. If, for example, someone's OCD consists of a fear of germs, then maybe the first step on their hierarchy would be the touching of a kitchen counter and not washing their hands for one minute. Once this was accomplished, their next step might be holding their hands on the counter for two minutes and refraining from washing for five minutes. After successfully completing each step, they then attempt the next one and hopefully, continue on until they reach the pinnacle of their hierarchy. For germaphobes, perhaps this summit would be performing a dumpster dive or touching the floor of a public bathroom without washing for several hours. The simplicity of describing such a hierarchy, however, belies the actual execution of its steps. It's one thing to talk about facing one's fears and an entirely different one to actually do it.

Several questions immediately arose concerning Ray's exposure hierarchy. How much input into its development should Ray have? Should he decide on the steps and write them out; should we negotiate on the steps; or should I just bull ahead and create the thing on my own? My suspicions were that leaving it up to Ray wouldn't work because inevitably, he would aim low. His entire hierarchy would most likely consist of baby steps that wouldn't take him very far. In other words, instead of moving upward towards a summit, his plan would probably take us in circles. And, who could blame him? Nobody wants to face their fears because it's a difficult and painful process. As for me, I had the opposite problem. If it had been up to me, I would have constructed a hierarchy that was almost perpendicular to the ground. Forget steps; let's just find a rocket to propel us to the top. But, I also knew that this gung ho approach would backfire; if Ray was pushed into facing too much, he would probably shut down and refuse to move at all. A delicate balance needed to be maintained between our two extremes if we were to achieve success. What I finally decided was to compose the hierarchy myself without much input from Ray but to remain vigilant to his stress levels. If it looked as if he was fraying in his resolve during an exposure, I would back down. If, however, it looked like he was sailing through, I would increase the pressure.

Ray also agrees that he shouldn't have had much control in designing the ERP. Maybe for others it would have worked, but for us, it was better for me to maintain control.

ΔΔΔΔ

One of the reasons my ERP worked so well in treating my sexual obsessions is because I had almost no input into creating the therapy. Thankfully, my mom never asked me for my input into the ERP. If she had, I know for a fact that my therapy would have been too easy and therefore, highly ineffective.

Many times, I would fake my symptoms in an attempt to trick my mom into creating an easier ERP exercise. I can remember, for example, being shown an image of a nude woman in a college sexuality textbook and then looking away quickly and putting on facial expressions that made it seem like I was more bothered than I was. Even though I had initially felt large amounts of anxiety when first shown such pictures, I had grown used to them. But, I still acted like they bothered me because I knew that if my mom had realized how easy that exposure had become, she would move on to more explicit exposures.

On occasion, my mom would ask me what kind of exposures we should do or what was really bothering me at the moment. I would often be too embarrassed to say what my thoughts were (as they were sexual in nature) or too scared to tell her in fear that she would make me face them. In fact, I cannot remember truthfully responding to any of her questions regarding what kinds of thoughts were bothering me at any moment.

For those who truly do not understand how effective ERP can be to ridding OCD of its power, they should not be given any control over the nature of their ERP therapy. When ERP was first suggested to me as a way to deal with my OCD, I would have bet my life that doing ERP would not make my pain go away but only exacerbate it. Thus, even though I was convinced to do ERP (mainly by getting paid to do it), I used all means I had to make the ERP easier on me. If I had been allowed to design my own ERP therapy, I know that I would have not gotten better.

ΔΔΔΔ

Another dilemma I faced was deciding if I should put the hierarchy in writing, like a contract. Maybe if we had such a contract, Ray would be more resolved to honor it or more hesitant to break it when the going got tough. My main concern with this idea, however, was the loss of flexibility in deciding what exposures to try. As anyone who has ever signed a contract knows, there is little room for negotiation after the signing. If exactly what was expected of Ray had been written down, I feared that he would use it as an excuse not to try new ideas that arose during the therapy. We would be stuck following a rigid plan when what was needed was a more fluid one. Fortunately, Ray never pushed hard for the details on his ERP plan, and I decided that it was best not to commit ourselves.

Our First ERP Session

Our first ERP session took place during the Christmas break of Ray's sophomore year of high school. He had been told beforehand roughly what was expected of him and how much he would be paid. We would work on ERP almost every day for several hours, taking Christmas and New Year's day off. I had debated on how much to tell Ray regarding the specifics of the ERP plan and had decided against telling him much. Even though my tendency is to explain my reasons for doing things, I worried that if we talked about ERP and its specifics that Ray would decide to back out at the last minute.

On the first day of our ERP session I felt nervous, like I was starting a new job that I wasn't qualified for and that at any moment someone would see me for the fraud I was and fire me. Ray mainly looked angry because he had to get up so early on his first vacation day to do this. If so much hadn't been at stake, namely Ray's future, I would have given in to the temptation to turn tail and run. I was that scared and felt that unprepared.

Ray's first exposure on the first day of the ERP session was simple: We would take turns reading out loud from human sexuality textbooks. I had found several of these books in the hallway of our local university's science building underneath a sign indicating that they were free for anyone who wanted to haul them away. My thinking at the time was that maybe these books contained information that would help me better understand sexuality and adolescent males, which I could then use to help Ray understand his sexual obsessions. There wasn't any compelling reason to start Ray's exposure in this manner; any number of ways could have been used since his OCD was triggered by the slightest hint of sexuality. We could have, for example, simply started by looking at pictures of females in a magazine, by going to a supermarket and walking around to watch women shopping, or by looking at pictures of female classmates in his yearbooks. Perhaps it was the multidimensional aspect of the material in the textbooks that caught my attention. These books seemingly had it all; from the dry, boring reading that is commonly found in most textbooks to explicit drawings showing nudity and sexual positions, almost what one might find in a pornographic magazine. For someone who suffers from sexual obsessions, the material in these books could fit nicely into many, different steps on their exposure hierarchy.

To get us started, I picked out and read a paragraph that hopefully wouldn't trigger Ray's OCD too fast and furious but would instead, ease him into the exposure. He looked anxious but survived the reading. For his turn, he took his time, and I suspected that he was looking for a paragraph that didn't address any aspect of sexuality. One would think that in a human sexuality textbook such paragraphs would be rare but in reality, Ray easily found and then read them out loud with enthusiasm. He did this because to him, these paragraphs didn't trigger any of his bad thoughts, and he could sail through his turn without feeling anxiety. During each time that it was my turn, however, I would search out paragraphs that were more difficult for Ray to hear. Any paragraphs that contained sexually-explicit words, such as sexual intercourse, vagina, penis, orgasm, or masturbation, caught my eye and were sure to be read. Ray, of course, hated this and on several occasions, accused me of purposely trying to make him mad.

Knowing if an exposure is working is an important part of successful ERP therapy. Without challenge and anxiety, an exposure can't work; it's nothing more than a walk in the park when what is needed is a strenuous workout. Within a short time, I learned to gauge an exposure's effect on Ray. If he readily agreed to an exposure, if he appeared relaxed before, during, and after an exposure, or if he remained talkative after learning about a new exposure, then I knew we had taken a wrong turn and had better try a different path. If, however, Ray grew quiet, showed obvious signs of anxiety like pacing, grimacing, or hand wringing, or immediately started arguing about the merits of an exposure, then I was sure our path was right and that it was wise to stay the course. During our paragraph readings, Ray's anxiety quickly elevated, indicating that this exposure had a good chance of working.

In addition to doing exposures, the other critical part of ERP is the prevention of compulsions. Exposing someone who has OCD to what triggers their obsessions but then letting them perform their compulsions is like running in place; you wind up exhausted from your efforts but have not gone anywhere. Since compulsions are performed in an attempt to lessen the anxiety caused by obsessions, it's important to prevent their execution during ERP. In fact, any act that lessens the anxiety that is experienced during ERP should not be permitted. In other words, initiating feelings of anxiety, letting them grow, and staying with them until they let up is the ultimate goal of ERP. With this process, someone who has OCD retrains their brain to let go of their obsessions and to demote those obsessions into normal, everyday thoughts. During Ray's ERP sessions, it was our goal to forestall, as long as we could, any of the several compulsions that he would normally perform, such as hand and feet washing, taking a shower, or confessing his bad thoughts. In the beginning, this was difficult because Ray's compulsions were a part of his habits. Ask anyone who has tried eliminating one of their bad habits how hard it is, especially one that gives them pleasure, such as smoking, eating certain foods, or drinking alcohol. Ray's compulsions were like bad habits and were ones that had given him pleasure because they lessened his anxiety. Adding to the problem was that Ray would automatically perform his compulsions whenever an obsession shot through his brain, which at one point, occurred as often as several times per minute.

My goal during our first ERP session was not the elimination of Ray's compulsions, that would have been expecting too much, like asking a three pack-a-day smoker to quit their habit overnight. Instead, we would chip away at the compulsions, delaying hand washing for a few minutes, using less soap (ie, fewer squirts of hand soap) per each washing, washing only hands and not feet, or delaying how quickly a bad thought was confessed. We didn't have a definite plan on how to do this. Prior to starting the ERP session, Ray had been told how important it was that he not do his compulsions, but I had not laid out exactly how we were to accomplish this, mainly because I had no clue how to do it. How do you prevent someone from performing an automatic act other than constantly reminding them or physically standing in their way? In the end, that's what we did; I policed his actions. Whenever he left the room, he was followed to make sure he wasn't heading towards the nearest sink to wash up; if he feigned needing to pee, he was monitored from outside the door and reminded about how much soap to use; if he confessed his thoughts, he was ignored like he had said nothing. At times, I even stood between him and a sink reminding him not to wash and for others, I watched a clock and reported on how many minutes had passed since he had expressed wanting to wash. We did whatever we could to disconnect the associations between his obsessions and compulsions.

On the first day, it was obvious that Ray needed a break from his ERP after our session on reading from the human sexuality textbooks. He needed time to decompress his ballooning anxiety and to regain his mental strength. If it had been up to me, we would have kept going, but I realized that Ray needed some control in determining the pace of his ERP. He knew his breaking point better than anyone and if pushed beyond it, there was a danger of him shutting down and refusing to start up again. What I did insist on, however, was that the breaks remain short. He was allowed to spend about an hour doing something pleasurable, such as playing a video game or going for a walk. But shortly after an hour, I would find him and remind him that it was time to start again.

For the second half of Ray's first ERP day, we did something a little easier: Watch TV. For a long time, Ray's OCD had restricted him to watching a limited number of shows or had caused him to change channels several times per minute. In fact, any program that had females present would trigger Ray's obsessions, which made it easy to find one to use as an ERP exercise. For these exposures, all we had to do was to turn on the TV and start watching whatever was on. Our goals during this exercise were to keep watching a program for as long as Ray could, to not change the channel (this one was easy because I maintained control of the remote), to have Ray stay sitting during the program and not get up so he could easily turn away, and to not confess any bad thoughts that arose during his viewing. One problem with this exposure, however, was that it was easy for Ray to cheat. He could, for example, simply pretend to watch but really avert his eyes from the program and not watch whenever someone came on that triggered his obsessions. My clue to this happening was when he acted too relaxed during our viewing. In other words, the exposure was going too smoothly for my comfort. The solution to this problem was for me to once again, police his actions, and to do this I watched exactly where his eyes were focused. If his eyes were anywhere but on the television screen, he was reminded to keep watching the program and that the whole purpose of the exercise was not to avoid anxiety but to feel it and push past it. Needless to say, Ray found this process annoying and didn't hesitate to voice his anger.

After the TV viewing, Ray took another short break, and we finished the day talking about OCD and its many components. Since Ray was too frustrated with me to listen to my thoughts on the subject or to hear anything that remotely resembled a lecture, we opted to read from several OCD books. My first pick was to read a chapter from *Imp of the Mind*, a book written by Lee Baer, where he specifically addresses OCD that manifests mainly by the presence of intrusive thoughts, such as sexual and violent obsessions. Ray was interested in listening to the descriptions of others who had similar obsessions as his own and how they overcame their fear at having such obsessions. Knowing that others had faced down the same demons and had lived to talk about it gave Ray hope that he could also do it.

Much to our amazement, we survived the first day of Ray's ERP without mentally breaking down, physically breaking something, or hitting each other. The temptations were there to give up, pack up, and concede Ray's life to OCD. But, we stayed the course and resolved to try again the next day. We spent the evening trying to recover our sanity and resume a normal existence. This evening, like many evenings during our ERP sessions, we got out of the house. Throughout all the sessions, we often went to movies, rented movies (Ray would have symptoms during these movies with the difference being that they were for enjoyment and not exposures; he was allowed to have his symptoms during these movies), ate a lot of cheeseburgers, consumed gallons of ice cream, drove around town for miles, and did whatever it was we could think of to have some fun. Ray would have preferred hanging out with teenagers his own age, but his OCD had caused him to lose most of his friends, and he wasn't up to try making new ones. At this junction in his life, I was not only his mother and therapist, I was also his only friend.

The other days of Ray's first ERP session went much like the first one. We kept reading from the human sexuality textbooks but made slight changes to the routine on almost every day. In other words, we kept moving up our exposure hierarchy. We went from having me to read the more difficult paragraphs to having Ray read them out loud, and once he was handling this routine without melting down, we graduated to viewing the drawings in the books. Ray had noticed these pictures on many occasions when he was searching for a paragraph to read and had commented on how anxious they made him feel. Admittedly, I wasn't comfortable viewing these drawings with my teenage son, but I also knew that any embarrassment I felt paled in comparison to the anxiety Ray was feeling. Even though the pictures were drawings and not photographs, they were vivid and detailed. By the end, we had viewed, reviewed, and then reviewed again drawings depicting every different sexual position two people could have. We also stared at numerous vaginas and penises in all states of health and development. As with the TV viewing, I did what I could to keep Ray honest during these exposures and watched his eyes as closely as I dared to make sure that he was looking at the necessary parts of the pictures and not lazily gazing at the innocuous parts like feet or hands.

We also stepped up our TV and movie viewing during our first ERP session to gradually include more sexually-explicit material. At the beginning of our session, we started with programs such as "Family Guy" and the Harry Potter movies but by the end, we had moved onto more risqué material. We spent hours at our local video store, looking for movies that contained variable amounts of sexuality, ranging from sexually suggestive to the depiction of actual sexual intercourse. The pinnacle of this exposure was when we viewed a movie, rated NC-17, which showed a scene of a young man with an erect penis hovering over a nude, equally young, lady. For the exposure, Ray not only had to watch this scene without standing up and leaving but had to watch it over and over again. I, with remote in hand, would rewind the scene to its beginning and repeatedly play it. How many times that scene was played I've long forgotten, but I do remember that Ray, after a certain number of viewings, had reached a tipping point. With each subsequent viewing after that one, Ray became less anxious and less needy of his compulsions for relief.

What Ray remembers from that first ERP session is similar to my memories. He does, however, have ideas about it that can only come from the one who is undergoing the therapy.

ΔΔΔΔ

I can easily say that ERP was the hardest thing I have ever had to do or ever will do. The amount of anxiety that I often felt during the midst of that first ERP session was indescribable, and I can remember several occasions where I would rather have ended my life than continue doing it. This description may sound exaggerated, but for me, these feelings of anxiety were very real and very strong.

When my mom first approached me with the concept of doing ERP, I was, to say the least, repulsed. She, in essence, was attempting to persuade me that by embracing everything I feared and hated, I could overcome my obsessions. This general principle made sense to me but at the time, she might as well have been asking me to overcome my fear of heights by jumping out of a plane without a parachute. This was how averse I was to doing ERP and accurately illustrates how much I wanted to avoid my fears imposed by OCD.

When I was finally persuaded to do ERP (with money as an incentive), I had a set plan in my mind to pretend to do the therapy. I would fake some of my fears and then do some "exposures" to convince my mom that I was doing the therapies in order to satisfy her and to keep me from having to do the exposures that targeted my actual fears. But, as I was to learn, she was prepared for this and quickly caught onto me and my plan.

Our first ERP session began with simple things like looking at sexuality textbooks and the pictures they contained. I cannot even describe the anxiety I felt doing these mild exposures. I remember clenching my fists as hard as I could and even holding my breath to somehow mitigate the anxiety that looking at those pictures provoked in me. I remember screaming at my mom and hit-

ting the walls around our house in an attempt to relieve some of those anxieties. The only things that kept me from running away during those exposures was my mom's relentlessness in keeping me focused and the short term rewards I was getting from doing them, but these things were only barely keeping me from giving up.

These exposures continued and every day for the first few days I dreaded waking up in the morning, because I knew I would be bombarded with the unrelenting anxiety that the exposures brought with them. Looking back, I would have given up if it wasn't for the twinge of hope I began to feel. After the first few exposures, I could feel that I was not getting as worked up about my obsessions. Albeit the anxiety was still high, but it was not at the pinnacle as it used to be.

ΔΔΔΔ

By the end of the Christmas break, Ray was more than ready to return to school. We had gotten through the two weeks of ERP relatively unscathed, and amazingly, we were still talking to each other and were even spending fun time together. Before we had started the ERP session, I had concerns that our relationship might be irrevocably damaged but had decided to take that chance, because ERP was something we had to do if Ray was to have an OCD-free life. What I had pushed Ray into doing in such a short time was difficult. I had made him face some of his worst fears and made him do it repeatedly for two weeks. If I had been Ray, I would have hated and resented me.

ΔΔΔΔ

After my mom and I had seen a therapist, who was supposed to help treat my OCD but ultimately failed, my mom decided to take things into her own hands. She admits that it was a risky move to con-

front my OCD on her own as my therapist while at the same time still having to be my mother. After all, at the time when I was struggling with my OCD I was like many teenagers and got easily frustrated at my mom and tended to disregard a lot of what she said about anything in general. I easily got mad at her, whereas I would hold back my frustrations and anger towards a teacher or therapist in the same situation. Therefore, when doing ERP therapy, it sometimes got very difficult.

This raises the question: Which parents are fit to guide their kid through ERP therapy? In my opinion, the answer to this question is simple: A parent should not have to be responsible for leading their kid through ERP. After all, parents take on a multitude of tasks, such as paying the bills, maintaining a household, and keeping track of all the things adults need to, and having to include ERP therapy into this mix is impossible. The reason my mom could pull off this herculean feat of pushing me to do ERP was because she gave up her full-time job as a pediatrician and devoted all her time to help me. If a parent is unable to devote a lot of their time to push their kid through therapy, then the struggle will be slow and painful and would be best left to a professional who can both efficiently and thoroughly conduct the ERP. If however, a parent can devote their time to understanding how to conduct ERP as well as implementing it, then I think that their kid will get better much quicker than if they saw a therapist for only a couple of hours a week.

Another pertinent issue for me regarding going through ERP with my mom as my therapist was how it has affected our long-term relationship. Today, I can discuss anything with my mom with no fear of reprisal or embarrassment because of the close relationship we developed going through OCD. During ERP, I often had to describe to her my worst fears. At the time, these fears were so bad that even saying them out loud made me anxious and scared, but my mom helped me get through it. Therefore, I have absolutely no fear of discussing anything with my mom. I can definitely say that having my mom as my therapist greatly strengthened our relationship to an extent that is unparalleled among my friend's relationships to their parents. Furthermore, because my mom guided me through my therapy, I no longer have to worry about OCD bothering me in the future because of how close she is. In other words, I do not have to worry about the availability of my therapist if my OCD should ever come back to bother me. She will always be there for me.

After the First ERP session

In the dustup that was Ray's first ERP session, neither Ray nor I could gauge what was happening. In other words, we weren't sure if it was working or if we were wasting our time. As the dust settled, however, and we looked over our new landscape, we were simply amazed. It was like a tornado had picked us up in some barren desert and then had set us down in a lush and vibrant forest. The difference in Ray's OCD was that great.

By the end of the first session, many of Ray's OCD symptoms had vanished, especially those symptoms that we had targeted during his ERP. He could watch many TV programs and movies without his obsessions gaining control; his need for reassurance had lessened; and his hand washing had markedly decreased. But, there was more. Many other symptoms, which had not been addressed during the session, were also gone. He was walking, for example, over floors in our home without worrying about contamination and jumping around like the floor was on fire; he was touching the TV remote and VCR buttons without first thinking about their cleanliness; and he was sitting on couches and chairs without asking about contamination. And the one that made my heart soar: He no longer flinched whenever I touched him.

Ray was also a different person outside our home. Before the therapy, he often acted like he was being hunted. Whenever he was in a building, he would slink along the side walls, ever vigilant as to who was in his vicinity, and if a female came close by, he would quickly change directions and walk away. If we were walking down the street and he saw that a female was walking towards him, he would become anxious and move away, sometimes even crossing the street. He would also often get up and change his seat whenever a female happened to take the seat next to him. After the first ERP session, however, many of these behaviors were gone, and he behaved more normally. We had not targeted these behaviors, but they had magically vanished anyway.

I will never forget the moment it struck me that Ray was different and that OCD was no longer completely in control. It was shortly after completing our first ERP session, and we had gone shopping at a local supercenter. I was braced and waiting for the usual torment that OCD was sure to cause. I was hurrying around throwing items into the cart, expecting that at any second, Ray would be agitating to leave because he was having too many bad thoughts about the females in the store or that he would be telling me that he was going to the bathroom, yet again, to wash his hands. Then, it dawned on me; Ray was not with me. This was unusual. Normally, he was close by so that he could either confess his endless thoughts or beg me to leave when the pain of his OCD got too overwhelming. Ominous feelings overcame me as I pondered this situation. Where was he? Was he cowering in some corner of the store because his fear had finally overpowered him, and he was now paralyzed? Was he stuck in the bathroom going through endless cycles of hand washing? I thought that maybe the ERP had backfired and that I had permanently damaged his brain. Like a mother who has lost her toddler, I panicked and started frantically searching. Relief washed over me when I spotted Ray in an aisle, standing upright, looking calm and normal. There was even a woman standing close to him, and he acted like he didn't see her. In a strange twist of thinking, I was tempted to tell him that she was there and wasn't he going to move away or run to the bathroom. OCD had so messed with my thinking that it took me several seconds to recognize normal behavior when I saw it in Ray. And, Ray was acting normal, not OCD crazed, but just like everyone else. He then turned, saw me, and smiled. It was all I could do to keep from dropping to my knees and thanking my lucky stars that I had found the magic bullet of ERP.

With mental disorders, such as OCD, it's difficult to quantify improvement. There's no blood test or brain scan we can have that tells us that we are getting better and by how much. After Ray's first ERP session, we both knew that he had gotten markedly better. At the time, I didn't try putting a number to that improvement; I was too much in awe of what had happened. In retrospect, however, it's clear to me that Ray's OCD had improved by a large margin, maybe even by as much as 50%. In other words, his OCD had backed down by half after the first ERP session. After this Christmas break and seeing what effective ERP can do, I even dared to hope that Ray would have an OCD-free future. If just one intensive session could accomplish so much, was it possible that multiple sessions could reduce his symptoms to close to zero? My enthusiasm for this idea, however, was tempered by one nagging thought: Would the improvements that Ray had achieved be retained in the long term or would his OCD come back, like a cancer that had initially been stopped by chemotherapy but had returned?

Once Ray restarted school after his Christmas break we didn't plan on doing any further ERP until his next break, which was three months away in March. Since our experience with ERP taught us that to do it properly requires intensive time, energy, and focus, we knew that trying to combine ERP with school wouldn't work. Either his ERP would fail, which would be devastating, or his grades would suffer, which would only add to Ray's problems. The question then was what to do in the meantime. Our options included doing nothing and hoping that Ray's OCD wouldn't regain its strength until we could restart the therapy during Ray's next school break; we could try mini-versions of ERP to see if what we had learned during our session could be miniaturized and used with smaller amounts of time, such as after school and weekends; or we could try a hybrid plan where Ray would be reminded of his symptoms when they appeared and encouraged, but not forced, to experiment with ERP to see if it could lessen his symptoms. After considering all ideas, we decided to take the third option. OCD, when and where it appeared, would be identified, and Ray would be given ERP-like ideas on how to push it back.

As the weeks trundled by I waited, hoping for the best, but preparing for the worst. With OCD, there is often disappointment and frustration, so imagine my wonderment when Ray's OCD showed no signs of growing but remained the smaller version of its former self. Here I was expecting our newly formed ground to give away but instead, it remained solidly under our feet. Through the first part of the spring semester, Ray's OCD remained mostly where we had left it after the first ERP session. It hadn't worsened, but at the same time, it hadn't improved either. This reinforced to us that for Ray, ERP was the main weapon we had against OCD. Whatever damage ERP had inflicted on OCD was real and long lasting, but it needed repeated applications to do more. It wasn't like an immunization that would keep working after just one shot; we would have to keep applying it.

Additional ERP Sessions

During Ray's spring break, we picked up ERP where we had left it after his Christmas break. This time, however, we only had one week instead of two so we had to adjust both our approach to ERP and our expectation for success. I wondered if seven days was long enough to accomplish a successful ERP session, but I also didn't want to waste the opportunity to try. We had considered waiting until Ray's summer break, but worried that too much time (six months) would have passed between sessions. I was concerned that our success from the first session might fade if we didn't quickly try the ERP again. Ray, as expected, wasn't thrilled to undergo ERP again but was persuaded (or bribed depending on one's outlook) to participate via a cash offer.

We started off the second ERP session by revisiting the human sexuality textbooks and having Ray review the pictures he so hated during the first session. As before, Ray was asked to look at drawings depicting sexual acts and to keep looking at them until his anxiety decreased by an appreciable amount. Because he had previously done this exposure and survived it, this viewing wasn't as hard as before. In fact, he sailed through it, which told me that he was ready to attempt the next steps on his exposure hierarchy.

One difficulty with planning the next exposures was how far to take them. When working up an exposure hierarchy, it's often difficult to decide how fast to move. One could, for example, take baby steps with each exposure only minimally more difficult than the last or larger and harder steps could be attempted. My tendency was often to reach for the sky and have Ray stretch as high as he possibility could. Ray, of course, preferred a more measured and slower pace. Resolving these two tendencies wasn't easy, but since I was in charge, it was usually my plan that was tried first. I also knew that if I was wrong and had overreached on an exposure that we could always retreat and start again where we had left off. Ray had showed me during our first ERP session that he wasn't fragile; he might bend some, but he wouldn't easily break. This experience gave me the confidence to try harder and more difficult exposures.

After our first ERP session Ray was better, but he still had OCD symptoms. There were still many things in our home that he couldn't easily touch; he still had difficulties whenever females were close by him; and there remained one bathroom in the house that he still decisively refused to enter. Life was better, but OCD was still too much in charge for my comfort. If we wanted to dislodge OCD from our lives, we would have to push hard during the second ERP session. But, how to do this? I had already used many of the obvious ideas, such as viewing sexually-explicit material in movies and having Ray look at drawings in the human sexuality textbooks. Most ideas that I had readily thought of for our second session didn't seem much more difficult than what we had already done. We could, for example, read sexually-explicit novels, not the sugar coated romance novels that are a dime a dozen, but more raunchy, sex-laden ones. When I looked to see if such material actually exists, I was flabbergasted to find that a whole genre has been developed in this area. Upon reading parts of these books in our local bookstore, I was impressed that writers had found ways to pack so much sex in so few words. But, I didn't think that these books would help Ray more than what the movies already had, and I also knew that he wouldn't read them on his own. I would have to read them, out loud to Ray, and I suspected that he would find ways to ignore what was being read.

The other idea I had was to take Ray places, such as malls or parks, where I would encourage him to look at females. This idea came about after reading about a priest, Father Jack, whose OCD consisted mainly of sexual obsessions. Once Father Jack understood that his obsessions were part of a clinical disorder and that to get better he needed to undergo exposures, he allowed himself to look at women and not worry about how he was viewing him. Using only this simple exposure, Father Jack's OCD quickly retreated. Father Jack's success with this exposure, however, succeeded mainly because he actively participated in it and repeatedly performed it on his own. He actively embraced it, which was far from the situation with Ray. Ray still needed pushing and cajoling to try exposures and required active enforcement to assure that he was participating in the exposures. Whereas I admired Father Jack for his approach in treating his OCD, I knew this approach wouldn't work with Ray.

One of the craziest ideas that I have ever had happened because of OCD and our ERP sessions. In looking for an effective way to set up Ray's new exposures, I realized that maybe we needed to try something more radical. Because we had already used the conventional ideas of sexuality for Ray's exposures, I decided to try using one of the more unconventional ones: Pornography. Even today, I'm still shocked that I considered using pornography as a therapy tool. My idea was simple; Ray would view pictures from pornographic magazines and do this several times a day for an entire week. I knew that many others would disagree with this idea, find it disgusting, and perhaps even disturbing, that a mother would do this activity with her teenage son. But, I wasn't going to let what others thought stop me. OCD had proven itself too wily an enemy to be defeated by conventional weapons. And, if I thought that I could save Ray by marching into hell, sitting down with the devil, and making him a deal, I wouldn't hesitate to do it. Would any parent?

The first step in setting up this exposure was to find some pornographic magazines. My plan was simple: Go into a bookstore or gas station, locate the magazines, march up to the counter, look the cashier in the eye, choke back my embarrassment, smile confidently, and make my purchase. The problem was that I couldn't find any of these magazines for sale. Stores either had sold out of them or didn't sell them at all. The closest I came was when I saw a distinguished looking, older gentlemen pick up the last copy in our local bookstore. I actually thought about asking him to give it to me, using the explanation that it was needed for therapeutic purposes.

Because my search in local stores had failed, I tried online stores and quickly found more pornography than anyone could view in a lifetime. The decision then came down to which magazines to buy and how many. This is when another crazy idea surfaced. Instead of diving right into the pornography that would trigger Ray's obsessions, maybe we could start with the type that wouldn't. In other words, the first magazine that we use should contain pictures of men instead of women. This way, Ray could get an idea of what to expect, like a dry run. Another advantage this way had was to let Ray see how I behaved when put under stress. Up to this point with ERP, he had borne all the stress and had been expected to keep pushing through. My role had been that of a coach who incessantly screamed from the sidelines and who was never satisfied with his performance. Maybe it was my turn to suit up and jump in. By doing this, I wanted to show Ray that his mother was willing to do whatever it took to help him and sacrificing a little dignity by viewing pornography seemed like a small way in which to do this.

Even after purchasing the magazines for the exposure (a copy each of *Playgirl*, *Playboy*, and *Hustler)*, I hesitated. I worried that the exposure could backfire and cause us more trouble than help. Maybe after viewing such material, Ray would develop negative ideas regarding women and their sexuality. The pictures in *Hustler*, for example, are outrageous, misogynistic, and unhealthy, and I wondered how Ray would view the women in those pictures. Would he respect women less after seeing such pictures; would his ideas of women's sexuality be skewed more towards the perverse, or would he understand that those images reflect only a minority's view on women? What I finally decided to do was to hold the more outrageous material (ie, *Hustler*) in reserve and start with the relatively more respectful (ie, *Playboy*). I still sensed that this exposure could work in ways that less controversial ones couldn't. I didn't know for sure, of course, but I was willing strike at Ray's OCD in whatever way I could.

What did Ray think when he was told about this type of exposure and how he was going to spend his school break? I remember extreme anxiety, anger, apprehension and even, disbelief that his mother would think up such an idea. What Ray remembers is similar, but he also now recognizes that it was an important step to take.

ΔΔΔΔ

Thinking about ERP therapy in hindsight, I have come to this conclusion: There is no level of absurdity that should limit what kind of exposures ERP should entail. For example, if someone with OCD has a deathly fear of germs, specifically those germs that reside in a toilet, it is not out of the question to work up to an exposure where that person would actually put their hand in the toilet (something a person without OCD would never do). What effective ERP needs to do is target a fear in any way possible and as intensely as possible, often by going straight to the source.

In regards to my OCD, I had terrible anxiety attacks relating to anything that was remotely sexual in nature. Even watching the Harry Potter movies (whenever any woman appeared and regardless of what she was doing) would trigger my anxiety because I would imagine some sort of sexual action in regards to any woman. At my worst, I could be doing absolutely nothing and suffer a bad sexual thought every ten seconds. Therefore, for my therapy, we aimed to trigger the most anxiety-triggering thoughts

172

possible. We started with simple sexuality textbooks and eventually, moved on to some of the hardest therapies that we ever did.

Looking at explicit pornographic magazines as a teenager with my mom, at first glance, seems ridiculous, maybe even perverse, but it was a vital step that had to be taken if my OCD was to be defeated. We had to trigger the most anxiety-invoking thoughts possible. Without invoking these apex thoughts, I might have been kept in fear, even if I had done exposures for all the other obsessions I had. Therefore, we did not consider that looking at explicit pornography was the wrong step for me. Many would disagree and think our exposures immoral, but for me, they served as an ugly means to achieve a happier end.

Creativity often comes into play when searching for therapies that can directly attack OCD. For example, I often had a fear that if I dropped anything on my pants, it would have come into contact with semen. I would then immediately try to get it off my pants without having to touch the object. For example, if a French fry fell on my lap, I would somehow try to brush it to the floor, and then I would have to pick it up with a napkin, throw it away, and wash my hands extensively. If I was nowhere near a sink (like on a car ride), I would just leave the object sitting on my lap until I could throw it away properly. During one of my ERP sessions, my mom and I targeted this obsession by deliberately dropping food onto my lap, then eating that food without washing my hands. As absurd as this exposure sounds it worked like a charm.

As a final message: There is no limit to how ridiculous an exposure may seem. If it can target an obsession, it is worth trying.

∆∆∆∆

When the time came to try using pornography as an exposure, Ray and I sat down, placed the magazine between us, and started paging through. The first round wasn't too bad because we had started with the *Playgirl* magazine. Ray was a little uncomfortable during this exercise but didn't express any major degree of anxiety. If anything, I was more uncomfortable than him but was careful not to demonstrate any distress. The next step (ie, viewing the *Playboy* magazine), however, was different. As with other exposures, Ray's anxiety upon viewing the pages in the *Playboy* magazine soared; he grimaced, vocalized his distress, stood up and paced, and tried to turn certain pages quickly so that he wouldn't have to look at what triggered his obsessions. My role, as before, was to keep him as honest as possible and focused on the exposure. I would often turn to the necessary pages of the magazine, remind him to keep looking at what bothered him and not at something else, and encourage him to look for as long as he could. I never timed these viewings, even though the idea had occurred to me. I figured that using a timer during exposures would have probably irritated Ray more than it helped. Instead, I used my judgment to decide how long each exposure was to last.

Using Ray's anxiety level as a guide, it was obvious that the exposures were intense enough to be effective. Throughout the week, we used the magazines for exposures during the mornings and used the afternoons for teaching sessions on OCD. We continued our readings from books on OCD and included some memoirs that had written by those who have OCD. My hope was that if Ray learned about the experiences of others who have OCD, that it would help him feel less alone and give him hope to see that others had overcome their OCD.

Even before our second ERP session had ended, I knew that our success wouldn't match that of our first one. Ray was doing what was asked of him, the exposures seemed intense, and he had seemed to habituate to the magazine pictures, so why wasn't it working like before? What was so different about this session that it failed to impact Ray's OCD like the first one? One possibility was that this session wasn't long enough. The first session had been conducted over two weeks instead of one, and maybe if we had had more time, we would have seen more results. The second possibility as to why this second session hadn't worked as well concerned the actual exposures. Even though Ray acted like these exposures were intense enough to work, maybe I had misjudged their impact or maybe they were too similar to our previous exposures to make a difference in Ray's symptoms. After thinking it through, however, I realized that the major reason for our lack of progress probably wasn't lack of time or the use of weak exposures. This time, the problem was me. I had failed.

Throughout our second ERP session, my performance was lackluster and not up to my usual standards. There were times when I didn't push Ray very hard during his exposures, and my vigilance during the exposures wasn't as intense, which allowed Ray to cheat more. Our breaks had also become more frequent and longer in duration, which caused us to lose momentum with the exposures. There was even a day when we gave up early and didn't resume the ERP until the next day. By the end of our session, all these factors had added up and as a result, Ray's OCD hadn't budged by much.

As with any team, success depends on the performance of all its members. When all members are in top form and working hard, good things happen: Games are won, projects are completed, businesses become profitable, and lives are saved. But when certain key members fail to do their jobs, failure is almost guaranteed. This is what happened to our team of two; Ray's ERP session failed because I didn't do my job. Where I had been in top fighting form during our first ERP session, I had acted passive, indecisive, and dull during the second one. The obvious questions that arose were why did I behave this way, and what can be done to prevent it from happening again? I have never found any good answers even after a lot of soul searching. I had hoped to identify specific factors that had led directly to my problems and that they were ones that could be changed and prevented from surfacing again. But, this didn't happen. The main conclusion I arrived at was that either laziness or tiredness had been why I failed to actively engage Ray's OCD for the second session.

My confidence in my ability to help Ray get over his OCD was shaken after not seeing good results after his second ERP session. Even with our remarkable success during Ray's Christmas break, I worried that a mistake had been made in having me conduct his therapy. Maybe our previous gains had just been the result of beginner's luck or maybe we had already grabbed all the low hanging fruit and that any additional success would require an expertise or nuance I didn't have. I was considering giving up the fight when I remembered that we didn't have many good alternatives. It was either give Ray up to OCD or to make another stand against it. So, I picked my sorry self up, brushed myself off, and started planning the next attack.

Dealing with a condition as nasty and tricky as OCD and then having its treatment equally difficult is like adding insult to injury. Conducting successful ERP is complicated, delicate, time consuming, and requires more creativity than most endeavors in life. Because of this, it shouldn't have been a surprise when the stumbles occurred during Ray's second ERP session. In fact, we shouldn't have felt bad at all. What we were attempting to accomplish requires a skill set that takes time to acquire and much practice to achieve proficiency. It was like we were being asked to design a complicated machine with only a ghost of a blueprint, road test that machine after building it, and then correct all its deficiencies before taking it out for a long road trip. With this thinking, the second session wasn't so much a failure but an opportunity to find the holes in our ERP plan and to patch them up before embarking on the next journey.

Final ERP Sessions

Using the experience we obtained during our first two ERP sessions, I started planning for the third one, which would take place sometime during Ray's summer break (between his sophomore and junior years of high school). Since our experience had taught us that two weeks was long enough to make a substantial dent in Ray's OCD symptoms, we decided to find two weeks during the summer and dedicate them solely to ERP. Like the previous ERP sessions, we wouldn't do anything but work on exposures as hard as we could. Initially, I had considered fitting in two or more of these two-week sessions during the summer but had finally decided against it. Two weeks of constant ERP is draining, both mentally and physically, and I didn't think that Ray would agree to give up even more of his summer vacation. I also didn't think that I had it in me to do more than one ERP session during this time.

During the several months between sessions, I had surveyed Ray's OCD symptoms and had picked out my targets, both large and small, and by the time our third session started, I had a long list of exposures to choose from. Ray's symptoms during this time had remained relatively stable, and he hadn't picked up many new ones. He was still fairly uncomfortable around females and remained wary of those objects and people that he thought had been contaminated by sexual material. There was one symptom, however, that had gained prominence since our last session. This symptom, which we had dubbed his "checking" compulsion, was one in which he would scan his body for any feeling or sensation that could be interpreted as sexual. And because he was looking for it, he often found it. To deal with his anxiety, he would run into the nearest bathroom and "check" his clothing, looking for evidence of sexual secretions and if he detected something, he would then engage in hand washing. Sometimes, he would look for me to confess that he had felt something. Other than this one symptom, however, his OCD hadn't gained much ground between our sessions, and I was hopeful that another round of ERP would knock it back even further.

For the third session, I added in some smaller exposures, such as touching certain doorknobs in our home without washing and becoming more comfortable with human contact. Even though these avoidances weren't high on our list of problem behaviors, they still caused us minor irritations, like a constant, but small itch that requires frequent scratching. You can live fairly well with it but would prefer not to. Prior to this session, we hadn't worked on these smaller problems, because I thought it was more important to work on the larger ones, an approach that I hoped would give us more bang for our buck. I also had hoped that most of these minor symptoms would melt away once we had tackled the bigger issues. Even though many of these small OCD behaviors had indeed disappeared without being specifically targeted, there still remained several.

One of the smaller symptoms we worked on was to have Ray touch certain doorknobs in our home. One doorknob, which particularly caused Ray problems, was the one that led from our kitchen to the basement where his room was located. For a long time, Ray refused to touch this doorknob with his bare hand and would either call me to open the door or use a barrier, such as a napkin or piece of paper, between his hand and the doorknob so that he wouldn't have to touch it. During our session, however, we didn't use a formal exposure to target this doorknob. Instead, I reminded Ray every time that he had to use the doorknob to please use it in a normal manner and not wash his hands. Since this door was in a high traffic area of our home, this happened multiple times each day. Another minor exposure we did during this session was to have Ray take items from my hand without worrying about how "dirty" my hands were. I had found this symptom particularly demoralizing and humiliating. Even though I knew it was the OCD and not Ray who was behind this behavior, there were times when I felt that my own son was looking down on me because he didn't consider me clean enough. The exposure for this symptom was simple: I handed Ray items throughout the day, sometimes even purposing brushing my hand against his during the exchange.

Another behavior that we focused on during this session was handling items that fell onto Ray's lap. For a long time, Ray would become anxious when anything, such as French fries, pens, or pieces of paper, fell onto his lap. He would immediately claim any fallen item as "dirty" and insist it be thrown out. Most of the time, this wasn't a problem, and I let Ray throw away the item. On occasion, however, the situation was more serious. I remember one instance when we were in a car, and I handed Ray my wallet so he could get some money. Upon opening the wallet, all my cards (credit, bank, and insurance) fell out into his lap. We both froze knowing what was coming: Ray insisting that the cards either be thrown away or be scrubbed into ruin. The situation was made even worse because we were in the car, and Ray couldn't just stand up and let the cards fall off his lap. He was in so much panic that he acted like he was being repeatedly stung or that the cards were on fire and burning him. He was also bouncing up and down and screaming at me not to touch the cards. If I had been thinking, I should have drove home, let him jump out of the car, run into the house to wash up, and promise him that I would scrub all contamination off the cards. But, I didn't. Instead, I stopped the car where it was safe to do so, insisted on gathering up my cards, and boldly declared that the cards were never to be washed. The effort this took was unbelievable. Once OCD takes control, it's almost impossible to defy it and in this case, I was stupid enough to try.

As with many exposures, we started our falling-on-the-lap exposure by doing something that would provoke a small amount of anxiety and then gradually, worked up to the most difficult. We started by placing food items, such as a potato chip or a French fry, on Ray's knee and letting it stay there for about thirty seconds. Then, Ray had to pick up the food item and eat it. Once he had mastered this step, we slowly moved the food items up his leg until they were close to his genital area. Each time, he was expected to eat the item and not throw it away. To keep Ray from escaping and washing his hands, we did this exposure while we were driving. The final step for this exposure was to have Ray place a food item high up on his lap, let it rest there for a while, and finally, hand it to me so that I could eat it. The success of this exposure was amazing, and by the end of the session Ray no longer reacted strongly when anything fell onto his lap.

During the third session, we also revisited the magazines that had been the bulwark of the second session. Even though there were questions regarding how effective that session had been, the high anxiety that Ray showed during those exposures made me suspect that it was worthwhile to attempt them again. We started these exposures at the same place where we had last tried them, that is, viewing pictures from a *Playboy* magazine. Ray quickly habituated to these pictures, and because of this success, I considered stopping these types of exposures. But, I also wondered if we could use them to push even further. Since our session was in full swing and Ray appeared strong, I pulled out the *Hustler* magazine that had been held in reserve. Instead of viewing tasteful pictures of nude women, Ray's exposures now consisted of viewing raw, rude, and disgustful pictures of adults engaging in sexual acts. Even now, it's hard to believe that we survived these exposures, but we did. Ray did well during these viewings, forcing his anxiety down from immeasurably high levels to ones that were merely uncomfortable. In other words, these exposures, as awful as they were for the both of us, worked amazingly well.

As we had discovered during our first two ERP sessions, there

180

are many ways to conduct ERP. We had successfully used several, different methods, and I was confident that what we were doing was effective. But, I also was always on the lookout for additional ways and had found one that we hadn't yet tried. Several books on OCD mention a technique where someone, who has OCD, tapes their voice describing a scenario that triggers their OCD. Then, they repeatedly listen to their tape until their anxiety decreases by about half. It has been suggested that this technique works especially well for those who have intrusive thoughts of violence or sexual matters. I had no idea if it would work with Ray but decided to try it. No point leaving this stone unturned after all the rocks we had already looked under.

During the third session we used three tapes. Most of the time I wrote the scenarios because I suspected that Ray wouldn't put in adequate material to trigger his OCD, and if I kept sending him back to put in more, we would have wasted a lot of time and energy. To get him used to this technique, we started with a simple scenario that lasted about thirty seconds. In it, I had placed words that were sure to trigger Ray's OCD, such as breasts, erection, and semen. As expected, he reacted strongly when he read what I had written and even exclaimed that I was severely demented to have written something like this. But, he dutifully taped his voice reading the scenario and repeatedly listened to it. What surprised me about this exposure was how quick his anxiety waned, especially after watching his initial reaction. It was the fastest drop from such a high anxiety level that I had seen happen with Ray. It was like going from a hundred mph to zero in a matter of seconds.

The remaining scenarios that we used were longer and more intense. Each time, Ray taped himself reading them and then repeatedly played each one until he was bored. We were careful to follow the suggested guidelines, such as making sure there weren't any reassuring phrases like, "I would never do something like that, or this is so crazy, it's not something I want ever to happen," were included. It was also important that Ray, and not me, record the tapings so that it was his voice he heard describing the scenes. Somehow, hearing one's own voice express the OCD triggers makes it more authentic and powerful. My main role in these exposures was to write them out (some books suggest that it's best if the person who has OCD does the writing) and then police Ray when he was listening to them. I would sit close and watch to make sure that he was listening and not daydreaming. At one point, he asked if he could surf the internet or listen to some background music while listening to his tapes. I saw these requests for what they were: Attempts to find ways to distract him from actually listening, which would lessen the impact of the exposure. There was no choice but to say no, tell Ray to sit down, and start listening.

The reason we stopped at three tapes was because it had worked so well. By the third one, Ray had to listen only a few times before it lost its punch, and it was obvious that additional listening wasn't needed. It's possible, however, that more tapes and more time might have been needed for this type of exposure if we hadn't already trudged through our previous sessions. In other words, if we had started with the tapes, it would probably have taken a lot more of them to get the momentum needed to make some real damage against OCD.

Ray has some additional thoughts on using tapes as a method for performing ERP.

ΔΔΔΔ

In my opinion, voice tapes were not the method that helped me the most. The main problem with this method is that for it to be effective, the scenarios should be written by the one who has OCD. However, I often found that I was reluctant to bare my soul and use detailed descriptions for my worst fears. In other words, I refused to do what was necessary to make this method really work.

To get around this problem, my mom put together the scenarios for me to record. Even though she knew me pretty well and could make good guesses as to what would trigger my OCD, I think that it would have worked even better if I had been convinced to write them out. After all, I'm the only one who really knew what my thoughts consisted of and what thoughts really bothered me.

Another problem with using tapes is that it is often hard to find the right combination of ideas to make it really work, at least for me. Recently, I tried using this method to help me deal with some worries about college. I was struggling over one of my school breaks with the possibility of me getting kicked out of school for some small action that I had done (nothing all that bad, but my OCD wouldn't let it go) and to deal with it, I wrote out a voice tape that laid out in detail the scenario that I feared the most. I described how I would be expelled from school and that I would be stripped of all my grades and credentials that I had worked so hard to get. I also laid out in detail the shame I would feel after being shunned by all my friends for being a college dropout, as well as the shame my parents would feel for raising such a failure of a son. I read this out loud many times and even rewrote it to include additional ideas, but it never helped me very much. My mom thinks that the reason it didn't work well this time was because I wasn't persistent enough with it. She thinks I needed to have gone over the material many more times for several consecutive days. But, I'm not so sure.

Based on my experience, I think it is better to use an ERP technique that targets physical compulsions. If you fear germs, for example, do therapy that prevents you from washing your hands, or if you fear that you have hit someone on the road, do not go back and check. In these cases, voice tapes might not be the best place to start. But if your OCD is the type that doesn't have obvious compulsions, then I think using voice tapes can be useful.

ΔΔΔΔ

The Holy Grail for the third session was one I originally doubt-ed we could manage: Having Ray take a shower in the bathroom he so hated. This bathroom was one that his OCD had been focused on for a long time, and many of his symptoms could be traced back to this very room. Ray's OCD had convinced him that this area had become contaminated with sexual material because he used to shower there when he was younger and freely experimented with his body (ie, masturbated). His OCD further insisted that the contami-nation was still present and that it was easily transferred between surfaces. In other words, anyone or anything that had contact with that bathroom was contaminated and was capable of spreading it throughout the house by simple contact. An example of Ray's cas-cading OCD thoughts regarding this bathroom is the following: "My mother used that bathroom and because she didn't wash the bot-tom of her shoes that means that wherever she has walked is now dirty. Because the floor has not been washed after she walked on it, it also is contaminated, so when my cats walk over that same area, they pick up the dirt and spread it wherever they walk or any sur-face they jump on. My mother has touched those areas and had repeatedly contaminated her hands so absolutely everything that she touches is unclean and should be avoided." Many times, I have pic-tured this bathroom like some sort of mother ship that was actively spewing out triggers for Ray's obsessions and that it's destruction would help us win the war. But, was Ray ready to tackle his obses-sions concerning this bathroom, and how we would know if he was?

During the third session, I noticed that something different was happening with Ray. He was moving up his exposure hierarchy much quicker because he didn't require as much time or encourage-ment to work through his exposures. In other words, we were blowing through my plan much quicker than I had hoped. For a while, I worried that maybe this was happening because the exposures weren't intense enough, but I didn't think that was the case. The other possibility was much more attractive: Maybe Ray's OCD was quickly getting better and if that was happening, maybe we could reach for one of the exposures that had always hovered close to the top of his hierarchy. I decided to go for it and have Ray tackle the "evil bathroom."

Like so many exposures before this one, we took it slow and started off with Ray stepping into the bathroom with me standing outside its threshold. Once it became obvious that Ray was doing well, I asked him to take several further steps in and approach the shower. Within a short time, Ray's anxiety decreased, and he progressed to touching items in the bathroom, such as the faucet, sink counter, shower door, and even the toilet lid. Next, he was asked to take the great leap: Taking a shower in the bathroom that had so plagued him. I don't remember the particulars from that day other than standing in the kitchen scooping peanut butter by the spoonful and eating it while listening to the shower run. I was close enough to listen to Ray's activities in the shower and felt confident that he was indeed in the shower and not just letting the water run while he stood outside with his clothes on. As the adage says: Trust but verify. When Ray stepped out of the bathroom and assured me that he had done the exposure, I believed him and couldn't have been more proud than if he had saved the world.

Our success with the third ERP session mirrored that of the first one. After the two weeks, Ray's OCD symptoms had backtracked by a large margin, maybe even by as much as 50%. There was much more he could comfortably do, such as touching things and people, and he even looked like he felt more comfortable in his own skin. In addition to all his other compulsions, his checking behavior was also much less prominent, which likely meant that he was no longer monitoring his body for sexual sensations. By the end of our third session, Ray's OCD symptoms had diminished by so much that I wondered if any mental health professional who evaluated him could even make the diagnosis of OCD but would instead, think he had some sort of "OCD tendencies."

The combined success of our three ERP sessions was such that Ray was no longer controlled by his OCD. He could function in the world without having extreme anxiety, and our home life resumed normalcy. Overall, he looked happier, stronger, more confident, and was now looking forward to his future instead of being imprisoned in OCD land. Even with all this progress, however, OCD still remained in control in certain areas, but these were areas that I was willing to concede for a while. Ray still wasn't completely comfortable with his body and his sexuality, and I suspected that he had yet to resume certain normal, heterosexual male pastimes, such as eyeing girls, talking dirty with his friends, or masturbating. Furthermore, he didn't want to talk with me about these personal aspects of his life, and I accepted his hesitation as normal. What teenage boy wants to talk to his mother about sexual matters? We decided not to actively try and take the remaining ground that was held by OCD. I feared that if we pushed too hard, we could cause more damage than good. If anything, we would approach those areas that remained held by OCD in a more cautious, passive, and indirect manner.

During Ray's Christmas break of his junior year in high school, he took a large step and assumed more responsibility for his ERP. Since his OCD had retreated into an area where I could no longer enforce any effective ERP, it was now up to Ray to take the reins and see what he could do. My role during this modified ERP session had been reduced to pitching ideas and encouraging Ray to follow through with them. Success or failure for this session depended entirely on Ray. He picked the exposure, the timing for the exposure, and the pace for repeated exposures. The overall goal for this session, however, was one that I had decided: Ray was to become more comfortable with his body. To accomplish this, I suggested that he try an exposure where he views himself in the mirror before taking a shower and explores certain body areas during his shower. In my suggestions, I didn't use explicit words or instructions because I knew that Ray was uncomfortable talking with me about certain things. Instead, I merely hinted at what he should do.

Because my role was restricted during this session and because Ray's OCD symptoms were now less visible to me, I couldn't directly judge how effective his attempts were. If asked, Ray would shrug and change the subject, an indication to me that I was no longer in the loop and that he was now mainly in charge of his therapy. But, I often knew when he had made an honest effort during his exposures because he would emerge from the shower angry and irritable, much like how he behaved when he faced his previous exposures.

Even though Ray wouldn't say much to me about these last exposures as he was undergoing them, he is now willing to write about these exposures and describe how he felt about them.

ΔΔΔΔ

The hardest exposures I ever did were the ones I did alone that directly targeted my sexual obsessions and fear of semen. It is incredibly embarrassing for me to write about this topic as it is taboo in many areas of our society to openly discuss sex, but I feel it is necessary to emphasize how this therapy pushed me to get over my sexual obsessions.

One of the key components to my sexual obsessions came from my fear of contacting semen. The reason why I had such an irrational fear is unclear, but it is clear that my compulsions, such as washing my hands, avoiding certain bathrooms, avoiding doorknobs, and not being able to normally walk on floors, all happened in an attempt to avoid my contacting semen. I also had obsessions that caused me to think that anything that was remotely sexual in nature could yield semen. For example, if I had a thought that was remotely sexual or could be slightly interpreted as sexual, I often worried it could have caused me to have an "emission of semen" and thus, I would avoid all contact with my pants. I would not touch things that had fallen on my pants, and if I did, I would immediately wash my hands, sometimes emptying whole dispensers of soap during one washing.

Because of my sexual obsessions and obsessions surrounding semen, one of the targets of my therapy was to end my compulsive behaviors that I used to avoid semen. To do this, I initially targeted behaviors, such as going into the bathrooms I feared and even ate food that had dropped onto my pants. After a few sessions of ERP, I was over much of my avoidance behaviors, but I still had obsessions surrounding contact of semen.

To deal with this persistent obsession, I decided to directly target my fear of semen, and the only way I could think of to do this was through masturbation. I accomplished this mainly during an ERP session during one of my school breaks. The anxiety this exposure created in me was more intense than anything I had ever felt before. But after a while, my fear subsided, and I no longer had an irrational fear of semen. The main way I got through this intense exposure, however, was to simply focus on the cash reward I was to receive at the end of the ERP session. Otherwise, I do not think I would have ever had the courage to give these exposures a try.

Some people may argue that these kinds of exposures go too far and that my mom should not have paid me to do this. However, during my worst time of OCD, I had not masturbated for over a year and a half (considered by most to be a normal function among adolescents). I did not want to go through the rest of my life fearing sex, because I knew that such a life would pre-

vent me from becoming a fully-developed person. Therefore, tak-
ing the necessary steps to push me into seeing sex as a normal
function was crucial to finally abolishing my sexual obsessions.

When to Stop ERP

When we started with our ERP sessions, I didn't have an end-game clearly in mind. We couldn't identify some final summit that upon reaching, we could plant our victory flag. Instead, we started on this journey, hoping that our final destination would place us in the vicinity of normalcy (ie, minimal OCD symptoms). And after each ERP session, we were coming closer to where we wanted to be. We were on the right path, seemingly to take the right turns.

As any parent does when faced with their child's diagnosis of an illness, I immediately asked: Will my child be cured of this disease? Wanting desperately to hear that OCD is curable I was disappointed to discover from many sources that no, OCD can't be cured, but can only be managed like other chronic illnesses. Diabetics, for example, aren't cured but are kept safe by daily doses of insulin and dietary vigilance, and epileptics aren't cured but can have their seizures minimized by the daily use of medication. And so it also goes for mental illnesses like OCD. Daily management is the goal, not absolute riddance.

When the idea of management, instead of cure, took hold I felt a profound sense of resignation. I had entered into this battle prepared to win, not to compromise. I wanted the unconditional surrender of OCD and not some 38th parallel line that I would always have to respect. I was to lose, the experts told me. OCD would always be with us; we could minimize it, but not destroy it like an antibiotic destroys bacteria or a chemotherapeutic agent destroys cancer cells. How was I to fight this war knowing that I could never fully win? Why not just quit now and save my resources to use in some other, more fulfilling endeavor? But as Ray's parent, I knew that quitting wasn't an option. To give up would mean that Ray wouldn't have a fighting chance to have a decent life. Even though I knew that OCD couldn't be killed and that I

190

would eventually lose this fight on some level, there was one thing that no one bothered to mention: Just how close could we come to winning and push Ray's OCD completely out of his life? Here, I realized, the choice was mine. I could lose by a mile or run such a fantastic and strategic race that the ending was a photo finish. With this idea in mind, I decided to push, pull, lie, cheat, spit, charm, claw, connive, hit, and kick my way through my son's OCD. OCD be damned, full speed ahead.

With each session, ERP got us closer to where we wanted to be. As I watched Ray's OCD fade into a shell of its former self, I decided to keep going as long as Ray showed symptoms and as long as our energy and creativity held out. I would not stop until either Ray was symptom free or we became so exhausted that we couldn't take another step. I knew, of course, that it was possible that some of Ray's symptoms could not be eliminated even with ERP, but I would exhaust all ideas before accepting that fact. In other words, we would persist in pursuing Ray's OCD until the very end of our resources. And if the time ever came when we reached the end of our rope, I was even prepared to tie a knot and hang on.

Ray's success after our ERP sessions was more than I could have hoped for and amazingly, we got there without exhausting all our energy and ideas. By the end of the sessions, I decided that Ray was in such a good place that it was safe to quit pushing so hard. I rarely saw an OCD symptom, and I concluded that most of Ray's behavior was no longer being dictated by OCD. Was he completely normal or in other words, had he been cured of his OCD? Of course not, OCD always find a way to linger and even to flare up on occasion. With a condition as complicated as OCD it's not possible to definitely know when it's safe to stop pushing. There is no blood test to run or brain scan to use that can tell when someone's OCD is gone and that it's safe to stop treatment. What I knew for certain, however, was that Ray's OCD had improved to the point where he no longer met the criteria for a diagnosis of OCD. He had entered into a remission. We knew that his OCD would return, but for the moment, it was essentially gone. Our responsibility now was to remain vigilant, scanning for any sign that OCD was trying to return and be prepared to fight it off like we had previously done.

Times When ERP Doesn't Work

There is no doubt that it was ERP that saved Ray from his OCD. If anyone would ask me what is the most important thing that one should do to deal with their OCD, I would not hesitate to tell them about our experience with ERP. And, we are not alone. The authors of several memoirs and other personal narratives on OCD also describe the powerful effects that ERP can have. What this means is that our experience with ERP wasn't unique; there was nothing special about us that allowed ERP to work better for us than it would for anyone else. But even with all the success that ERP can have against OCD, there are still times when it fails or when it isn't even used in the first place. Why this happens isn't always clear, and I suspect the reasons are many and varied.

One reason that ERP isn't always used to treat OCD is because there are some in the mental health profession who think that ERP is too harsh and who advocate that other more gentler ways should be used. Some of these professionals claim that those who have OCD can "think" their way through OCD by changing their relationships with their obsessions. Some have even written books on this idea, where they have presented data and have made strong arguments for their methods. Whenever I read these books, I often have pangs of guilt because they suggest that I had made Ray un-needlessly suffer through his ERP. Did I make him go on a forced march without food or water when we could have been strolling in a park? I don't think so. If these methods were as effective as advertised, wouldn't they now be the standard of care for OCD? They're not. By far, more books on OCD and more OCD professionals point to ERP as the way to go.

Are there times, however, when a milder, more reflective approach to dealing with OCD is helpful and even better, than ERP? Even someone as ardently in favor of ERP as me can agree that there are instances when other interventions can work better. There are even some memoirs written by those who have OCD that provide detailed descriptions about how they overcame their OCD, not by the grueling path of ERP, but by a more measured, thoughtful, and less ugly approach. The reasons for why this approach works for some but not for others likely includes such variables as degree of OCD severity, age when treatment is engaged, and type of OCD. It's hard for me to imagine, for example, that someone whose OCD is like Ray's initially was could sit down and accept the idea that their OCD can be thought through. Their minds are too busy rewinding and replaying their endless obsessions for anything else to register. I also think that age is important because adults, who have more life experience and more of their frontal lobe on line (frontal lobes are the brain areas where judgment and planning mainly take place), can more readily accept the ideas that are represented in a purely cognitive approach to treating OCD.

ERP was the most powerful tool we used, but even I have to admit that there were a few times when it failed. Fortunately, these times were few and were mainly when Ray's OCD was mild and not threatening to turn into anything ugly. What we learned was that these minor OCD flares were small enough that other, more portable tools, than ERP could be used. As far as weaponry is concerned, ERP forms the heavy guns in the OCD treatment arsenal and is most useful when heavy bombardment is needed. When Ray's OCD was at its worst, we needed these heavy guns and used them every day and as often as we could bear. Entrenched OCD is like a large mountain that needs to be brought down, and ERP forms the cannons that can be repeatedly fired at it. With persistent bombardment, most OCD mountains eventually weaken and fall. But when OCD is mild and looks more like a foothill than a mountain, the heavy guns of ERP are ineffective. The targets are now too small for the big guns and something smaller, and more easily handled, is needed. Instead of ERP, techniques like refocusing or pure cognitive reasoning might work better.

One example of when ERP failed to help Ray occurred during his spring break in his freshmen year of college. During this break, Ray had an OCD flare, which lasted only about twenty-four hours. He had been out with friends doing what college boys mostly do during spring break: Hanging out and having a few beers. On one evening when it was time to go home, he didn't think that he should drive because he had had a few beers, even though he felt fine. His friend volunteered to drive him home but then realized that Ray's car had a stick shift, and he didn't know how to drive that kind of car. To get home, Ray decided to drive a few miles with his friend riding with him. Nothing happened, both arrived safely, and Ray's friend left. Within a few minutes of his friend leaving, however, Ray's OCD immediately took hold, and he began obsessing about the whole incident. He worried incessantly about what he had done, that is, driving when he had initially decided that he shouldn't. The main trigger for this flare, Ray later determined, was a comment made by another one of Ray's friends. This friend had wondered out loud why Ray was driving when he had already made the decision not to and had asked a friend to drive instead. This one comment had set off Ray's OCD.

After a short time of wrestling with his thoughts alone, Ray called me. The anxiety in his voice, the repetition in his words, and the constant reassurance seeking reeked of OCD, and I told him, even during that first phone call, what I thought this was: An OCD flare. Ray agreed but still couldn't let it go, and the thoughts continued to swirl in his head. He obsessed over the fact that he had driven even though he felt that he shouldn't have, that his judgment wasn't perfect, and that the possibility existed that something bad could have happened. Repeatedly, he wrestled with these thoughts, calling me several times over about twelve hours.

My first impulse was to reach for ERP to help Ray deal with

this situation. I suggested that he use imagery or tapes to play out the feared scenario. I thought he could imagine or talk about causing a bad accident where people, including young children, were killed and about how he would be arrested, lose his place in college, and spend the rest of his life rotting in jail. I also told him he should add something about me turning away from him and that he would be forever alone, without friends or loved ones to support him. We even tried minor versions of ERP by repeatedly saying some of these ideas out loud. But, Ray didn't find these ideas helpful. For effective ERP to occur, it has to arouse anxiety and the more intense, the better. But no matter how we phrased or enlivened his fears, the real anxiety wasn't there. In other words, his OCD was making him anxious but not to a large degree. And without this critical level of anxiety, we couldn't find a way to make the ERP work. It was like the OCD target wasn't large enough for the ERP guns.

What finally worked for this minor OCD flare was to simply have Ray refocus his thoughts away from OCD and toward more normal ones. He decided to rejoin his friends the next day and to continue enjoying his spring break. He said later that by being busy and talking with others that the OCD had backed off and had quickly quieted down. He learned that by not feeding his OCD thoughts, they left him alone. In other words, he stopped thinking about his obsessions, and they went away. It was a pleasant surprise for us that something as simple as refocusing Ray's thoughts had worked so well. Here I was bringing up the big guns when all he needed was a hammer.

Here Ray describes another minor OCD episode (his latest) where he found a way to deal with it other than using ERP (in spite of my trying to implement it).

ΔΔΔΔ

From time to time, my OCD will attack me in ways that are difficult for ERP to help me with. For example, during my most recent winter break, I was plagued with thoughts that involved the possibility of me getting kicked out of school. These thoughts arose after I let a friend use some laboratory equipment for personal use. I began obsessing that if someone had found out that I let my friend do this, then I would get in trouble. Specifically, I worried that I would get kicked out of school, stripped of my grades, and lose all that I had worked hard for. I went to extreme lengths to make sure that there was no evidence left in the lab and spent hours rationalizing all the reasons why I would not get caught, and why even if I did, I would not get in trouble.

These thoughts were bothersome. On some days, I would wake up each morning and the first thought I would have would be, "I just want to get this day over with so that I can go back to sleep and be free of these thoughts." The sad part is that at the time I was obsessing the worst, we were on vacation in Peru, and I ended up wasting some of my vacation worrying instead of having fun.

I thought: "This is obviously OCD, shouldn't I just use ERP to free myself of these thoughts?" So, I tried, again and again. I wrote out long and painful scenarios that explored the worst consequences of my actions. I challenged myself constantly with the idea of losing all of my friends, family, and opportunities due to my careless actions, but no matter how many times I did this therapy, I never felt better. Was I not feeling better because the ERP was not strong enough, or maybe I was not doing it often enough? I think one answer lies in the fact that there was no solace or comfort I could run to after I did the therapies. When I did ERP against my sexual obsessions, I could take a break by watching a movie or playing a video game to allow myself to relax. But because we were on vacation, I didn't have access to those activities. Also, because we were away from home, I couldn't do the ERP activities as often as I might have had we been at home.

When the ERP wasn't working, I next tried pure cognitive rationalization in the most complex of forms. I would rationalize to the smallest detail why my thoughts were ridiculous. For example, I would think about ideas similar to these: "It has been seven days since I let my friend use that equipment, therefore, there is no way I am going to get in enough trouble to be kicked out of school because I would have been notified by now." But no matter how much cognitive rationalization I used, I was still spending a lot of time obsessing.

After I had exhausted ERP and cognitive therapy, I tried meditation and through meditation I found my solution to dealing with these thoughts. I read about Tibetan philosophy and employed several meditation techniques to relieve my obsessive thoughts of their strength. Whenever my thoughts would arise, I would sit down (usually somewhere quiet if possible) and focus on being either completely still or on the silence surrounding me. After about five minutes, most of my anxiety was gone, and I could experience the same thoughts without feeling anxiety. I felt acceptance and happiness. In fact, the more I meditated, the less power my thoughts had. I would focus on letting the thoughts flow through my head but would not allow them any power.

A metaphor I often use for meditation focuses on imagining my consciousness as a sky, and the things that I see or think are the clouds. My mind becomes the sky, and my thoughts become the clouds; the clouds are simply there, never completely obscuring or bothering the sky. They are just floating by.

ΔΔΔΔ

These experiences reminded us that the multiple and various stages that OCD morphs into require different approaches. In some cases, a simple cleaning out of the mental debris is enough to sweep away the OCD. These are also the situations when the commonly-heard advice can actually work: "Just stop thinking those thoughts; go out with your friends and have fun, take a walk and clear your head; read a book; take a break." If we're lucky, Ray's OCD will stay where these simple maneuvers can work, and we won't have to dig deeper into our arsenal. But, I plan to stay prepared, keeping the big ERP guns well oiled and ready to use at a moment's notice. I know better than to ever let my guard down and be caught unprepared.

Pitfalls When Trying ERP

Even though we became firm believers in ERP, we understand that others haven't been so lucky. Why ERP works so well for some but not for others is not well understood and probably results from several, different issues. Even I can concede to the idea that ERP is ineffective for some who have OCD, but I suspect that in many cases, the reason why ERP fails is that it wasn't applied correctly. And after conducting ERP, I can identify several areas where ERP can easily go wrong. ERP will fail, for example, if someone's exposures aren't well tailored to their OCD or if their exposures aren't of sufficient intensity.

ERP will also fail because of a lack of persistence. Doing effective ERP is not as simple as facing down one's fears once or twice or dealing with them over one to two years; it takes multiple exposures over a relatively short time to work well. How often someone who has OCD prematurely gives up on their ERP is not known, but I suspect that it happens fairly often. Someone gets their OCD diagnosis, miraculously gets to a therapist who uses ERP, starts the therapy, but then quits when the going gets tough. Hopefully, they find their way back to ERP and become believers in its effectiveness. I wonder, however, what happens to the others who don't. Do they believe that ERP failed them and refuse to try it ever again? I know that if we hadn't repeatedly and doggedly pursued Ray's exposures, then it wouldn't have worked well for us. Persistence was definitely one reason for our success.

Another barrier to effective ERP is something that isn't often mentioned: Shortly after embarking on ERP, someone who has OCD might actually feel worse and not better. It's like being prescribed a medication that suddenly makes you so violently ill that you wish that you had just taken your chances with the original illness it was meant to treat. ERP does this; it makes one feel worse for a time before it kicks in and works its magic. It makes sense that this happens. Dur-

200

ing ERP, someone is asked to face their worst fears and to not do the only thing they know that will help lessen their anxiety (ie, their compulsions). It's like asking someone to stand in a downpour without using their umbrella and stay there until the rain finally stops. Their first impulse is to avoid getting wet by reaching for their umbrella (ie, performing a compulsion) but instead, they are asked not to use their umbrella and to get wet. And, only after they have gotten soaked and the rain has stopped (ie, their obsessions have ceased) will they start to dry out. My advice for anyone who experiences this initial downturn after starting ERP is to don't despair; in fact, it might be a good sign telling you that your approach will work. Keep going, don't quit, and have faith that if you stick it out, it will soon get better.

A third problem area for effective ERP is the development of the exposure hierarchy. For ERP to work, one needs a well-constructed and personally-tailored hierarchy. It's definitely not a situation where one size fits all. In other words, an OCD therapist can't simply pull up on their computer a detailed protocol for treating a particular type of OCD symptom. Everyone who has sexual obsessions, for example, can't be successfully treated via the same exposure hierarchy. Instead, each one needs their own, personal hierarchy in place if ERP is to work well. Where this can become problematic is in situations where someone refuses to reveal very much about their OCD symptoms. In our case, Ray would often refuse to talk about his obsessions because they caused him too much anxiety. When directly asked to talk about his symptoms, Ray would either answer in monosyllables or would only shrug his response. How could a therapist construct a good hierarchy in situations like this? Most of what they could put together for someone like Ray would be based largely on guesswork or second hand information that had been gleaned from loved ones. I suppose that such a hierarchy is better than nothing, but it would not be one that could efficiently help someone overcome their OCD.

One of the advantages of me being Ray's therapist was that I knew him well, and where this was especially useful was in the formation of his exposure hierarchy. He didn't have to tell me what bothered him because I already knew from watching him. This information also allowed me to construct a more fluid exposure hierarchy. This fluidity was especially important during the times when either an exposure was too intense and Ray was on the verge of giving up or was too mild and looked like it didn't have the punch to do very much. In these situations, I could quickly substitute one exposure for another and not have to completely stop an exposure to fix the problem. It was like having the necessary toolkit and repair materials on board an airplane and rarely having to ground it for repairs. Another way to think about this is instead of having twenty or thirty discrete steps on Ray's hierarchy, we had hundreds of smaller steps with each one similar, but not identical, to the one next to it. This formation gave us an incredible amount of flexibility in directing Ray's ERP.

Part IV – Additional Ideas for Treating OCD

Hank: An Unusual Therapy Aid

Ray's OCD story is not complete until we describe one important character: Hank. In fact, much of our success in beating back Ray's OCD can be contributed to Hank. He stepped in and saved us in more ways than we can tell. We have not introduced this fellow until now because to tell his story intermixed with the telling of the other parts of our OCD story would have been too confusing and may have even lessened the significance of Hank and what he did.

First of all, let us explain that Hank is not a person but an entity that was constructed to help us deal with the most difficult parts of Ray's ERP therapy sessions. He gradually took form sometime during Ray's first therapy session and eventually, reached his mature and final form during the subsequent sessions. Even though Hank doesn't have a physical form, his persona is loosely based on a living creature: A house cat. During Ray's first therapy session, I struggled with handling Ray's extreme anxiety, many times losing my patience and letting Ray see my frustration. As anyone who has dealt with ERP well knows, this therapy is fraught with pain, resistance, and reluctance. Many times, Ray balked during an exposure or loudly expressed his discomfort, actions that mentally wore me down. I started to break, often yelling back at Ray, stomping away from him, or expressing my disappointment that he wasn't working hard enough. Needless to say, these behaviors on my part were harmful and threatened to derail the whole ERP process even before it had time enough to work.

It was sometime during our struggles in the first ERP therapy session when one of our cats, Hank, jumped into my lap and quietly purred. I remember thinking how calm this creature appeared even though there was a storm raging around him and how his presence had a relaxing influence on me. It was funny, but with Hank in my lap, I was less quick to express my impatience. At one point, I thought about how wonderful it would be if Hank could speak and guide both Ray and me through our difficulties. I wondered if Ray would listen to him at those times when he couldn't listen to me. At those times when I had blown it with my intensity, nagging, and general stupidity could another voice help us get through? I had often desperately wished for another presence during some of our most difficult times, especially one that also intimately knew us, knew our history and everything that had previously gone on. It was like we needed another me but one who possessed a differently personality. I wondered if I could bring Hank to life, then maybe he could infuse us with his calmness and help us get through our ERP sessions with less drama and conflict. I don't remember the exact moment when this happened, but sometime during our initial ERP session Hank found his voice and expressed it through me. What his first words were has been long forgotten, but their effect was immediately felt and represented the beginning of a long and fruitful relationship.

The creation of Hank wasn't the first time I had separated myself into two different personalities in an attempt to help Ray handle his OCD. Prior to officially starting our first ERP session, I had tried using my doctor credentials (ie, pediatrician) as a way to bolster my credibility with Ray and to convince him to listen to me. After all, don't we listen to our physicians and do what they say? If I wasn't talking to Ray as his mother but as a physician, maybe my words would have more effect. I did this one day by "introducing" myself to Ray as Dr. St. John and by explaining to him that during my years in medicine I had helped many patients with both mental and physical disorders. I even used the same approach in questioning Ray like I had often used when seeing patients. Ray listened for awhile but then decided that my being his "doctor" wasn't going to help much. I didn't know at the time why Ray felt this way, but he later mentioned that this idea failed because he had little faith in doctors. The ones he had reached out to had not helped him and had not tried to understand his OCD. But even though our experiment hadn't work out, I did sense from watching him during this exercise that it might work in some other form. I just didn't know at the time what other form to try.

With Hank working through me, it was like I had an ally in our fight against OCD. Even though Hank's words were essentially mine, he was different from me, and Ray responded to him in ways he wouldn't to me. It helped, of course, that I was very careful to keep Hank separate from me and to not confuse our two personalities. Where I often expressed anger and impatience, Hank was a bastion of calmness and patience; where I used force during Ray's therapy, Hank would coax and use gentle persuasion; and where I would express my disappointment when Ray faltered during an exposure, Hank provided encouragement. In many ways, Hank was my opposite; he provided the carrot, whereas I wielded the stick. Maybe this is why he worked so well. With Hank working alongside me, I had access to two different approaches and could use whichever one we needed at a moment's notice. There were times, however, when I wondered if Hank's approach by itself could have been strong enough to guide Ray through ERP, but I don't think so. Even though Hank's calmness often helped, there were many times when Ray responded quicker to my pushing.

To keep my personality from intruding onto Hank's, I created a new voice and even had Hank speak with an accent. His grammar and rhythm of speaking was different from mine; he often mistakenly used plural instead of singular forms and would draw out certain syllables. He even had certain expressions that he routinely used and were ones that I rarely ever expressed. I made Hank's voice as distinctive as my limited abilities would allow so that there was never any confusion as to who was speaking. Since I have no acting talent, it wasn't always easy for me to conjure up Hank at a moment's notice, but I got better at it the more I attempted it and by the end, Hank would emerge the second he was needed. On occasion, he might even finish a sentence I had started.

It's not easy to describe who Hank really is, but one generality of his being is certain: He represents the best of us all. He's definitely the quintessential grandfather in that he always has time to talk, take a walk, or just be present. His wisdom is so deep that it could only have come from living a long time, and he always seems to know the right things to say. His patience is endless; he can wait for as long as it takes for you to open up to him. You even can treat him in the worst possible way, but he never holds a grudge and will simply wait for you to realize your error. He laughs easily, loves stories, and relishes his food (his only real vice). He loves all things natural, can work all day in the hot sun, and has amazing physical strength. In short, Hank represents our version of the most perfect being we could imagine, maybe not the ideal that others would construct, but ours, and since he was our creation, we were free to give him those qualities we most needed.

Another important attribute Hank had and one that was critical to his helping us was that he was asexual. Even though Ray's OCD centered on sexual matters, Hank never addressed any personal issues on sexuality. This helped us the most during Ray's most intense exposures where he was viewing pictures or listening to sexually-explicit material. With Hank sitting by his side, and not me (as his mother), Ray could steady himself and keep going with the sexually-laden exposures. Why this worked so well; that is, using a character for support whose sexuality is nonexistent was not clear to me at the time. But in retrospect, I think it worked because Ray's OCD had not only caused him to fear all aspects of sexuality but had also targeted me. I was his mother, so obviously, I had some experience with sexual matters and even though Ray never told me that his obsessions had latched onto me, I suspected that, at least on some level, my presence was a trigger for his OCD. But with Hank in charge, that trigger was essentially eliminated, which allowed Ray to focus more intensely during his therapy.

I was once told by an OCD therapist how he thought it was "creepy" that a mother had helped her son deal with sexual obsessions by using sexually-explicit material as exposures. Not surprisingly, this comment shook me up and caused me about a day's worth of intense worry. Maybe I had done something terribly wrong even though the therapy had worked amazingly well, and Ray's relationship with me was still strong. After thinking about it, however, I did get the therapist's point; it's not normal or healthy for a mother and her son to view such material together. Instead of recognizing the viewings for what they were (ie, ERP exposures), I could see how others would worry that some sort of pathological sexual excitement might have occurred during the therapy. Maybe even some on level, Ray was aware of this possibility, which is another reason why Hank's presence was so helpful. As for me, my mission during all this was to knock back the hated OCD, and I never once, felt any sexual feeling during our therapy, and it never occurred to me that others would think otherwise.

I never knew beforehand when Hank's presence would be needed but learned to immediately bring him forward when necessary. Ray and I would be talking about something, usually OCD related, and would suddenly be spiraling away from each other. Most of the time, our problems had been sparked by something I said that Ray found annoying or he would have detected an irritation in my voice. It was during these times that Ray would quickly shut down, and nothing I could do or say would get through. If it was possible to let the conversation die, I would let it go, but on many occasions our spiraling had begun because of an OCD-related problem. If I had left it up to Ray to decide when we could talk and deal with his OCD, we would have never worked on it because he would have avoided it in any way he could. It was during these times that I turned to Hank to get us through the barrier and hopefully, resolve whatever issue was at hand. Even if we couldn't resolve our problems, at least Hank would allow us to speak respectfully to each other and to amiably part.

Ray also thinks that Hank was critical in helping us through the many aspects of his OCD.

ΔΔΔΔ

Hank is undoubtedly hard to describe but without doing so, it would leave out a good portion of my treatment. Hank is, at essence, a spiritual being that my mom and I fabricated to make my ERP therapy sessions easier. At the time my mom and I were doing ERP therapy, we would often run into barriers. Instead of listening and doing my exposures, I would get angry, remote, and unwilling. My mom and I have decided that the reason for this apathy lay in the nature of the parent-child relationship during the teenage years. Many kids go through a phase where parents are often seen as oppressors, which results in kids ignoring almost anything their parents say. This thinking made our therapies hard because not only I was feeling anger towards my mom as she tried to get me to do something I hated, but because she was also my parent, and my teenage mind told me to ignore her. Once we discovered the powerful abilities of Hank, however, the situation quickly improved.

During some of our earlier ERP sessions, my anxiety levels would peak, and I found it too strenuous and hard to continue without some sort of comfort. To placate some of these anxieties, we often had one of our cats (named Hank) sit with me. Hank had an incredibly calm demeanor and often his presence in a room was enough to get me to calm down and continue with my therapy. When my mom would push me into a therapy exercise that generated too much anxiety, we would use Hank as a catalyst to get me going by personifying him as my therapist. When my mom acted as the therapist herself, I would only get angry, but when she played Hank as the therapist, I could find the calm to keep going. Because of this, Hank became my spiritual guide through my ERP therapy.

One of the richest examples I can remember that accurately reflects Hank's power was during the times when I had to vividly describe my bad sexual thoughts to my mom. She needed to know the nature of my thoughts so we could learn how to target them. But, for me to explain them out loud caused such anxiety that it almost served as an ERP exercise by itself. Naturally, describing out loud to my mom (or to any human therapist for that matter) about my obsessions that I had possibly molested someone or had experienced a sexual "emission" was awkward and thus, I would leave out parts that were too hard for me to describe. When my mom would catch on to this sidestepping, she would immediately revert to Hank's character because he was someone I was much more willing to describe my thoughts to. This way, we bypassed a large amount of uncomfortable feelings and kept my ERP therapy going.

Even during my most irate and irrational times, my mom could get through to me through Hank. During the midst of especially hard times, for example, when I was not supposed to wash my hands following an exposure, I became so upset at my mom's prodding that I felt nothing but absolute hatred towards her. At the time, I hated my mom as much as I hated OCD because of how much she was pushing me to do the therapy. There were even times when I did things as awful as slamming a door in her face. However, once she reverted to Hank's voice, I was able to listen to her and eventually get the therapy done.

ΔΔΔΔ

Hank not only helped Ray deal with his OCD, he also helped me in many, different ways. For one, Hank often bought me more time when dealing with an OCD-related issue because Ray had patience with Hank that he never had with just me. Even when Hank didn't have an immediate answer to an OCD-related problem, Ray had faith that he would eventually find the needed solution. Ray was also more willing to discuss the difficult parts of his OCD with Hank, which allowed Hank to gather much more information than me (ie, as me) and gave him more flexibility in solving Ray's problems. A second way in which Hank helped me was that he allowed me to be more creative. By invoking his presence, I had access to a whole different dimension in my thinking. As Hank, my mind was more open and creative, which allowed for solutions to our OCD problems to form easier. I think this happened because Hank's presence allowed us access, like a key, to a calmer place. And when we were calm, we could think much better than if we're stressed and under pressure.

Yet another way in which Hank helped me was during the times when I most needed to apologize to Ray. Simply saying that I was sorry after committing some horrible mistake wasn't enough for Ray to forgive me and to continue on with our therapy or with whatever else needed to be done. The best example of this happened one day when I was particularly frustrated with Ray's OCD and its endless requests for cleaning. Shortly before we needed to leave home for Ray to attend a class, he decided that his entire bedding was dirty and that I needed to wash it all, even though it had been cleaned just a few days before. He had gathered it all up and was headed for the washing machine when I stupidly tried to stop him by standing in his way. I don't remember why I did that; maybe the endless pain and anxiety that OCD causes had gotten the better of me and had temporarily overtaken my senses. What happened next was predictable. Ray pushed past me, even knocking me to the floor, and ran to the washing machine where he stuffed his sheets and whatever blankets he could into it. Instead of calming down, I only made the situation worse by pursuing Ray and yelling at him. How we ever got out of the house, into the car, and down the road to Ray's class I don't know, but it probably involved Ray's desire to get away from me.

During the time when Ray was in his class, my senses returned, and the realization that I had made a horrible mistake slowly dawned on me. But, what could I do? I could apologize but that probably wouldn't be enough. Maybe, however, Hank could help me and deliver my apology for me. By the time Ray's class was over and he returned to the car, I had left and Hank was now sitting behind the wheel, smiling, and holding a bag of cheeseburgers. As Ray ate, Hank explained how very sorry I was and how OCD had taken its toll on me just like it had on Ray. Ray listened to Hank and then mentioned several aspects of my behavior that he particularly found unhelpful and how he sometimes felt that I didn't understand how OCD had affected him. With Hank doing the listening and not me, Ray opened up and told him more than he could tell me. Ray could also hear and accept my apology through Hank's words.

Ray once asked me if I thought that having Hank involved in our lives was childish and that maybe he should find a way to deal with his OCD without his imaginary friend. Because we had become so dependent on Hank and his help, I immediately dismissed that idea. I saw no good reason for us to abandon Hank. Maybe Ray thought differently, but I had never thought that Hank's presence in our lives was abnormal. Even if we don't readily recognize or admit it, we all use fantasy in our lives and use it daily. The books we read, the movies we watch, and the music we listen to often serve to transport us away from our realities and lets us explore places, relationships, and ideas that would otherwise not be available to us. In fact, researchers have now suggested that over 50% of our awake time as adults is spent fantasizing about other ideas and people. It has also been proven that fantasy, in the form of play, is critical to the development of children's minds and in forming their problem solving skills. So much of what they dramatize in their play is not fun and games, however, but often the very fears that they have, such as abandonment, loss, and death. By playing out their feared scenarios, their minds learn how to handle these difficult life situations. If such magical thinking is so important in creating our adult minds, it makes sense to me that it can also serve as a creative way for us to solve our problems. And, Hank certainly helped us manage Ray's OCD in ways that no other source could have.

Having Hank in our lives and helping us through Ray's OCD was such a godsend that it made me wonder: Why haven't I heard about this technique before? Of all the books that I have read on OCD, both by the professionals and by those who have OCD, the idea of using a character like Hank is never discussed. The only time I ever heard about someone creating something similar was in a short article that was published in the International OCD newsletter and was written by a mother whose little girl had OCD. In the article, the mother described several fairy-like characters that she had developed to help her daughter understand and deal with her OCD.

The closest that the professionals come to advocating the use of imaginary characters is when they suggest that those who have OCD actually name their OCD. The basis of this idea is similar to why we developed Hank in the first place: The separation of identities. Where we used Hank to separate me from my mother-self, the naming of OCD allows those who have it to separate themselves from their OCD. In other words, with this technique, the OCD is singled out as a separate entity and is not considered an integral part of someone who has it. This helps during therapy because all negativity can be directed towards the OCD by name and not towards an individual. When a therapist says, for example, "I think your life would be better if you stopped listening to Mr. OCD and find a way to get rid of him," it works better than if you had just been told that OCD was ruining your life and that it was time you did something about it. Somehow, this separation allows one to think that their OCD really isn't so ingrained in them. Instead, it's a separate entity that can be cast off without having a devastating effect.

When Ray was younger we named his OCD and had found it helpful. (We have decided not to include our name for Ray's OCD in this book because some might find it offensive. For the purpose of demonstration, we will refer to Ray's OCD as Mr. OCD.) Using a separate name for Ray's OCD helped us in several ways, such as allowing us to address Ray's OCD behaviors in an indirect and less personal way. ("I know you really didn't want to ask me for the tenth time if it's OK for you to have your bad thoughts; it's Mr. OCD's fault because he's the one putting those thoughts in your head.") It also helped us to redirect Ray's thoughts away his obsessions to more healthy ones. ("I know Mr. OCD is making you think those thoughts that bother you so much, so why don't you stop listening to him and let's go have some fun.") I also invoked Mr. OCD after those situations when I had lost my patience and had yelled at Ray for something OCD related. ("I'm not yelling at you. I'm yelling at Mr. OCD for making you think those thoughts and not letting you be happy.") In addition, having Mr. OCD around was cathartic; he served as our punching bag because we could hit him whenever we felt overwhelmed by OCD and not feel guilty. He was also a good way for us to openly demonstrate our hatred of OCD and for what it was doing to our lives. Many times, we ritually killed Mr. OCD by any way we could think of such as stabbing him, setting him on fire, throwing him off a bridge, stomping on him, or choking him. These thoughts might seem violent to others, but they demonstrate how much hatred OCD invokes in those who have to deal with it.

When Ray got older and his OCD got more intense, we found that it was no longer helpful to refer to his OCD as Mr. OCD. This technique, even though useful when Ray's OCD was mild, failed to help when his OCD worsened. Because of this ineffectiveness, we gradually stopped using the name and now haven't used it for a long time. I also can't imagine the situation where we would use it again; presently, I refer to Ray's OCD as simply "your OCD or your OCD pathways" whenever I need to tell Ray that his thinking is starting down an OCD path. ("I think maybe your OCD pathways are involved because you have told me about ten times how you think you failed that test.")

Ray remembers Mr. OCD well and has this to say about him.

ΔΔΔΔ

By naming my OCD (Mr. OCD), it was easier for me to get angry at it. If my OCD was tormenting me relentlessly, I would immediately imagine some sort of entity named Mr. OCD who was solely responsible for making me feel horrible. By naming my OCD, I was able to acknowledge that what I was feeling was because of OCD and was not because of something that was real.

I think that one reason why many people who suffer from OCD do not get over it is because they are not convinced that they have a mental disorder but instead, feel that they are terrible and weak for having such strange thoughts. I felt this way for a long time. My sexual obsessions made me feel terrible, and I would blame myself for having these thoughts. For a long time, I thought that I was a horrible person and a sexual deviant because I didn't understand that these thoughts came from my OCD. My mom saw this in me and knew that the first step to getting over my OCD would be to convince me that my thoughts were a product of OCD and not a flaw in my moral character. By separating out my OCD and naming it, it made it easier for me to understand this important idea.

ΔΔΔΔ

After having Hank in our lives, I have concluded that everyone should have their own, personal Hank. We all need such an entity that we can turn to when our lives are in turmoil or when we need access to other dimensions in our thinking. Maybe for some, their religion can serve this purpose, and I admire those who can use religious teachings to help them through their difficult times. There are many accounts where this has happened, and I encourage anyone to follow this path if they are able. For others, however, the path is less clear, and the creation of a character, such as Hank, might be helpful.

I have no special formula to give others which tells them how to create their own Hank. There is no step by step process that if followed, would guarantee the production and functioning of another Hank. My best advice for anyone who thinks that this idea could work for them is to first think about perfection and the qualities that word brings to mind. Loyalty, patience, wisdom, persistence, humility, creativity, humor, courage, steadfastness, forgiving, and unconditional love are all words that leap to my mind whenever I think about Hank. He has all these characteristics and has honed them to a perfection that I will never achieve.

Of all the things Hank taught us, one of the most important was that we can use our imagination and creativity to solve the most difficult of our problems. Before Hank, I had never dreamed of using imaginary characters as a therapy tool, and even now, I can't say exactly how the idea came to me or how I had the courage to try it. But we did, and it has made all the difference. And, it worked so well that Ray and I didn't stop with the creation of Hank. We made others. In fact, at one time, we had a virtual community of characters that we often used to help us navigate through our lives.

When Ray's OCD had been fought back and we were taking stock of our lives, it occurred to us that we had become isolated. We no longer had friends that we could count on and our family connec-

216

tions had become too strained. We needed a community to help us rebuild from OCD, and since we didn't have access to a real one, we created a virtual one. Each of the characters we created served a unique role and could be called upon to help us deal with specific problems or to help us understand the behaviors of others. When Ray was feeling like he had lost all his social skills, for example, and didn't know how to speak to others, we would invoke the one character who could talk to anybody about anything but not care what others thought. His swagger, extroversion, and confidence represented the very skills Ray needed to develop. Another character we developed was one that was often anxious and initially kept asking if he was bad because he had done something. Eventually, he got over his "OCD," (once Ray understood not to constantly reassure him), but he maintained a low level anxiety about the world. Nevertheless, this anxious character found his niche and gradually become an invaluable part of the community. Many of our characters have flaws, make mistakes, and get into trouble, just like people do. We even create new characters when the situation calls for it; one of the latest was a very upbeat, nonstop talker, and eternal optimist called Sunshine who was brought to life during a time when Ray was depressed and couldn't shake it. Whenever he refused to talk to me about what was bothering him, I would send in Sunshine, and Ray would usually start talking (mainly so she would stop jabbering at him).

Many would probably scoff at our virtual community or feel sorry for us that we even created one. Even I admit that at times, our characters have a cartoonish patina and a silliness that is childish. But on a deeper level, many of them represent useful psychological principles that therapists use in their practice; through our characters we present the same ideas that a therapist would in a more professional setting. The goal of therapy is to change a patient's thinking from negative patterns to more positive and useful ones; for example, someone with depression who routinely thinks that he is a loser is encouraged to challenge that thought and to think of areas where he is successful. Or, maybe someone who feels that they are too shy to ever have friends is taught how to be more assertive and how to manage a conversation. Our community of characters serves the same functions for us; they show us different approaches to a situation, and we then decide which one would work the best. Many times, when faced with a problem, Ray would ask how each of our characters would handle that particular situation. On most occasions, he could walk away with a good solution and on those other times when the solution wasn't as clear, at least he felt heard, validated, and supported.

Medication - Our Experience

To medicate or not: This is a question most people (or parents) don't ever have to wrestle with. For most conditions, the benefit of medication is obvious. If someone's skin is dripping pus or if they're sneezing nonstop, they have no problems taking an antibiotic or an antihistamine. In fact, they would be viewed as odd if they didn't take these types of medications. And, no one ever questions the parents who willingly allow their kids to be injected with powerful drugs (eg, chemotherapeutic agents or anti-epileptics) if their kids need it. So, why are those of us who have a mental illness (or whose kids have a mental disorder) often questioned or even berated when we turn to medications? And, why don't we always feel comfortable when we do make the decision to use medications for our or our kid's mental disorder?

Ray took medications for his OCD when it was at its worst. In fact, our first contact with any mental health professional was with a psychiatrist, who readily prescribed Prozac, one of the several selective serotonin reuptake inhibitors (SSRIs), for Ray. I supported this decision and had even actively lobbied for it during our first visit. Ray's OCD had gotten so bad and was not showing any signs of letting up that I had no choice but to turn to medications. No other therapy could possibly penetrate the whirlwind that OCD was blowing around Ray. Even if we shouted, our voices couldn't be heard over the storm that OCD was raging in Ray. He could no longer hear anything else but what OCD was telling him. At this time, I could think of no other option but to throw a pill at Ray, hope he agreed to take it, and wait to see if his OCD winds died down. In our case, we hoped that the medication would act like a lifeline, which we could then use to hang onto Ray until we could pull him to safer grounds.

Prozac worked for Ray but did so suspiciously quickly. Many times, we had heard that the SSRIs can take up to six weeks before they exert their effect and that many doctors wouldn't consider adjusting doses until that time period had passed. Why it takes so long for these medications to work is still not clear, but most likely results from how the brain responds to these medications. This response includes such activities as slowly upregulating and/or down-regulating the levels of neurotransmitters (the chemicals the brain uses for communication) or their receptors (the structures that grab onto a neurotransmitter and hold it in place long enough for the transmission of messages). Some studies have also suggested that the SSRIs function by stimulating the birth of new brain cells (neurons), which then need time to grow, mature, and become wired into the existing brain network. Also complicating this issue is that the many SSRIs don't behave exactly in the same way. Even though they are similar enough to be included in the same class, they have differences, which result in them acting slightly different-ly and needing different time periods before showing their effects.

Ray's fast response to Prozac could have resulted from sever-al different ways. For one, he could have responded to it because he wanted to or had expected that he would. In other words, he had a placebo response; he could have been swallowing a green M&M and had the same positive response that he had to the Prozac. Several studies have suggested that for many medications, the placebo re-sponse is as high as 30%, that is, close to a third of people have a good response simply because they think they are taking a medication even when they aren't. Was this possibility something I worried about? Not really. Whereas I understood that for some medications a place-bo response is problematic, I didn't think it was a concern for Ray. Any improvement in his symptoms at this point would have caused me to drop to my knees and thank my lucky stars. I would have taken any improvement we could and not worry about the package it came in.

Many who have taken medications for mental disorders

know the long list of side effects that come with them and have experienced more than one such wayward effect. Ray was no different in this regard; he felt slightly nauseous, dizzy, had headaches, and felt jittery when he first started taking Prozac. And, he most likely experienced one of the most common side effects the SSRIs cause: Sexual dysfunction. Adults, who are given these medications, often throw them away, refuse to ever take them again, and try to find another way to deal with their condition all because the pills have taken away sexual desire. Life doesn't have many pleasures for some, so giving up the one activity that is guaranteed to generate pleasure is not something they are willing to do. But in Ray's case, having this side effect probably helped his symptoms. Because his obsessions were sexual in nature, anything that affected the physical workings of sexuality was bound to dampen his obsessions. The medication might have eliminated all his physical sensations of sexual desire that his OCD had always convinced him were wrong and were something to feel guilty about. As a result, he felt less anxious.

Even though the Prozac (for whatever reason) visibly helped Ray deal with his OCD, it didn't do nearly as much as we had hoped. It's hard to estimate how much better Ray was after taking Prozac; my best guess was that he was only about 10% better. But when someone has the huge number of symptoms that Ray had, even a little improvement feels miraculous. With Prozac's help, I felt that Ray had been lifted onto a ledge and was no longer dangling off a cliff with only a small rope to keep him from falling. That said, however, he was still very much in danger of being blown off the ledge with the next stiff wind.

Hoping to build on the initial help that Prozac gave Ray, we increased his dose, crossed our fingers, and waited. Weeks went by and nothing happened. His symptoms stayed right where they were, stubbornly refusing to retreat any further. Ray's psychiatrist then decided to give up on the Prozac and switched him to Zoloft, another one of the many SSRIs. Why Zoloft was picked next (and why Prozac was initially chosen) and not one of the other SSRIs was not based on any good scientific data, but instead, was mainly a best guess. Ray's doctor could have easily just written the names of all the SSRIs on a piece of paper, pinned them to a bulletin board, closed his eyes, winged a dart at the board, and wrote a prescription for whichever SSRI name had been speared. Ray's doctor wasn't being negligent or hopelessly out of date with regards to his decisions; it was because of the current state of psychiatric medicine. There isn't enough data, especially in kids, to help doctors make good decisions. Instead, they rely on their personal experiences and on their best guesses.

Switching from one SSRI to another isn't always as simple as closing one door and opening a different one. For some lucky people, it's easy; they suffer no withdrawal symptoms and can stop and start their medications as needed. For Ray, however, switching from Prozac to Zoloft was like trying to travel without following a road; in other words, it was very bumpy. And, we had an additional concern: There was no guarantee that the switch would make any difference. In fact, there existed the possibility that Ray could lose the little ground that Prozac had helped him gain. In the end, Ray decided to gut it out and after about a week of nausea, headaches, dizziness, and extreme irritability, he started feeling better. As for his OCD, there was no obvious change after his withdrawal symptoms had abated, but at least, it wasn't any worse.

Added to the concerns about taking medications for OCD is the fact that many psychiatrists use doses that are much higher than those recommended for other conditions, such as depression. Where someone might be given 50 mg of Zoloft, for example, for treating their depression, someone with OCD might be told to take upwards of 300 mg. What these mega doses are doing that lower doses can't is still a mystery. Personally, I'm not even convinced that such high doses are really effective. OCD is tricky; for some people it can come and go on a whim, and they never know why. If someone was taking a high dose of an SSRI when their OCD waned, it's possible that they and their doctor would attribute their improvement to the medication even though they were getting better on their own. If this happens to enough people, then the idea of requiring higher than usual doses to treat OCD could gain traction. And with little data to help doctors find their way, it's likely that such observations might be given more weight than they should. But, I will also admit that if Ray's OCD had ever retreated at the same time that he was taking a high dose of some medication, I would have kept going with it and not rocked the boat. I might not have liked it, understood it, and maybe even have worried about what such high doses were doing, but I would have accepted it.

The minute Ray's psychiatrist suggested that Ray sidestep to a different SSRI, I lost hope that medications would make a large dent in Ray's OCD within a short time. Because it takes up to six weeks before a certain medication at a certain dose is deemed effective or not, it can take a lot of time, maybe years, to find a workable combination of medicine and dose. But even with this in mind, we gave Zoloft a try, hoping that luck was on our side and that this medication would work. It didn't. Even after we had pushed Ray's Zoloft dose through the roof, his symptoms stayed at the same spot where Prozac had left them. No loss, but no gains either.

Now what were we to do? Here was Ray on a near maximum dose of Zoloft, and his OCD symptoms were still interfering with his life. Should we push the Zoloft even higher? Should we try yet another SSRI and if that one didn't work, continue our march through each one until Ray had tried every SSRI? Ray's psychiatrist even suggested that Ray could take a combination of medications, such as an SSRI and one of the newer antipsychotics. In addition, a quick internet search revealed even more ideas, such as taking two

SSRI's together and using medications (eg, d-cycloserine and clomipramine) that are not commonly prescribed for treating OCD. When I was done thinking about all this, my head was swirling. There were too many options, too many opinions, and not enough data. My son's life was at stake, and the only guidance I could find was based on guesswork. Where were the well-researched protocols that exist for other conditions, such as cancer, diabetes, or epilepsy? Why, instead of finding definitive recommendations for drugs and their doses, the best we could find was suggestions? We needed a well-defined map to get somewhere important but all anyone could give us was vague directions like, head north for a while, turn slightly left when it feels right, then go straight until you see large tree........You get the point.

When Ray's OCD stayed stubbornly entrenched after several months of increasing doses of Zoloft, I decided not to pursue the medication route any further, but instead turned to other treatments, mainly exposure and response prevention therapy (ERP). I understand that others might have made a different decision and continued searching for the right medication or combination of medications. And, I accept that for some with OCD, medications work well and have saved them from living an OCD-infested life. For Ray, however, medications weren't quickly working out, and so we decided to hold Ray's Zoloft where it was, thrown ourselves into doing ERP, and see what happens.

Ray's response to ERP was more than we ever dreamed. After each ERP therapy session, his OCD was pushed further back. The ERP was doing what we had originally hoped the medications would do, that is, make Ray better. As Ray fought his way to mental health via ERP, we wondered what to do about his Zoloft. Should we keep it on board at his current dose; should we try lowering it and if we do, how fast should we go; or should we forget it and have Ray stop cold turkey? We decided that immediately stopping Zoloft wasn't a good idea for Ray; he had previously undergone significant withdrawal symptoms when he switched from one SSRI to another, so we assumed that he would have similar symptoms if he were to quickly withdrawal from Zoloft.

Keeping him on his high Zoloft dose also didn't make sense. Why should he continue with a medication that we didn't think was helping? Also, all medications have risk; some are known, but a lot are unknown and are only discovered years after being in use. I worried that one day a researcher would report a previously unknown and deleterious side effect that shows up mainly in those who have taken high doses of Zoloft. I had nightmares of reading headlines like, "Zoloft now shown to increase incidence of brain tumors, or early deaths detected in those who take high doses of Zoloft." Even though this scenario is unlikely, after all, the older SSRIs have been around for over twenty years and have been taken by millions, I still didn't want to take any unnecessary chances, especially where my child's brain is involved. Of course, I wouldn't have worried much about what Zoloft was doing if it had been helping; I would have been thankful for whatever benefit it gave Ray.

After we decided to take Ray off of Zoloft, the next step was figuring out how to wean him from it. Ray's psychiatrist let us figure out how to do this and for that, I was grateful. Since our previous experience with weaning Ray from an SSRI showed us that he was sensitive to changes in doses, we knew that he would have to go slow, taking baby steps over a long time. Instead of having him wean off his Zoloft within a couple of weeks, we would take months. The other decision we had to make was how to integrate Ray's Zoloft wean with his ERP therapy. We had several options: Wait until he had finished with most of his therapy before lowering his Zoloft; attempt to wean while he was undergoing an ERP therapy session; make changes only between his sessions and not during one; or forgo any consideration of integration and follow a defined schedule for weaning. Another question I had was this: Was it possible to use the Zoloft wean in a way as to augment the effectiveness of his ERP therapy? We had learned during our first ERP session that anxiety, as terrible as it feels, is an important component to successful ERP therapy. In fact, for Ray, the more anxiety he felt during a session, the better results we had. In other words, the more pain that Ray felt during his ERP sessions, the more gains he made. Perhaps this seems awful, and even counterintuitive, for those who have little experience with ERP therapy, but for us veterans, it's law.

When I noticed that Ray would become irritable and mildly anxious after a Zoloft wean, I decided to use those feelings as a running start to his ERP sessions. Instead of easing ourselves into a session, we would be charging into it. Ray's brain would already be primed to handle the anxiety and maybe he could use it to propel him through the therapy. Did this strategy work? To my thinking, it did. Ray hated it, but several days before each of our ERP sessions we would decrease his Zoloft dose, wait for the withdrawal symptoms to appear, and then plunge into the therapy. By the end of the session, he would often have markedly less OCD symptoms and would also be one step further along on his Zoloft wean. Even though this strategy worked for Ray, or at least didn't derail his therapy sessions, I realize that it might not work for others. For some, the anxiety caused by withdrawal symptoms combined with the anxiety of doing ERP therapy might be overwhelming and in that case, it would be better to forgo any medication changes and instead, focus on the therapy.

With each step downward in Ray's Zoloft dose he would feel it for several days. He would have slight nausea and mild headaches with dizziness. But, none of these symptoms were too harsh for Ray, and he continued on. Only when he reached about the halfway mark did he get inpatient and decide that he wanted to try coming the rest of the way off in one large step. Instead of stepping carefully and slowly picking his way down off his Zoloft mountain, he decided to jump the rest of the way. He knew it would probably be a hard landing, but he would be down. I agreed to let him jump, not because I thought it would work, but because he was insistent on trying it his way. By this time, he was so sick of being told what to do that he wanted control of something, and this was one area where he could call the shots. After all, no one could force him to take the pills; even if I had refused to agree to his plan, he still had the last word because he could refuse to swallow his Zoloft.

Within a few days of taking the plunge, Ray regretted it. His withdrawal symptoms fired up with a vengeance, and he was hurting. He knew he had made a mistake but wasn't sure what to do. Should he try waiting it out, knowing that eventually, he would feel better, or should he return to where he last felt good? I had no advice for him. It was like watching him dangle by a rope halfway down a large cliff. He could climb back up to safety, which would put him right back where he had started, or he could cut himself loose and hope he landed somewhere safe. Either choice wasn't great. For a while, he kept waiting it out even though his symptoms remained intense. But when they persisted and started to affect his school performance, he decided to go back and start over. We returned his dose back where it had been and waited for his symptoms to abate. Ray had hoped that by dutifully returning to where he last felt normal that he would quickly resume his normal functioning. It didn't happen. For a couple of weeks he remained sick, luckily not as strong, but still bad enough that he didn't want to do much but stay home and sleep.

Once Ray had finally returned to baseline and vowed never again to attempt large steps in his Zoloft wean, we devised a new plan and returned to using small, incremental dose changes. But, even that plan didn't work out as well as we would have liked. With each change, his withdrawal symptoms were strong, interfering with school and with his already-diminished social life. The other problem he faced was that the symptoms now stayed and refused to budge like they had before. At times, Ray wondered if he should go back up on his Zoloft because he was feeling so bad for so long. It seemed like he had reached a critical tipping point and that it would require much more effort than before to decrease his Zoloft. This situation reminded me of people who want to lose large amounts of weight. The first twenty or thirty pounds come off easily, but then it becomes much harder to drop the last ten pounds.

To make the final push to come completely off Zoloft, we had one final visit with Ray's psychiatrist. We did this mainly because Ray needed a prescription for Zoloft pills which were of a smaller dose than the ones we already had. It was like we needed a small screwdriver to get a job done, but all we had were large ones. With the new pills, we had the tools to lower his dose in very small increments. Even with this plan, however, Ray still had significant symptoms. They were not as bad as before, and he was able to gut it out until he finally reached his destination.

With each step downward, we not only waited out the withdrawal symptoms but also waited to see what Ray's OCD would do. We knew that it was possible that we had been wrong about the Zoloft and that it was doing more than we realized. Perhaps all the credit we gave to Ray's ERP therapy for pulling him through was unjustified and that the Zoloft had been holding an important key all along. Maybe our plan to wean Ray's Zoloft would backfire and that his symptoms would come raging back once the Zoloft was gone. Maybe I had done something really stupid like giving away my beloved guard dogs because I naively thought that all threat was gone. This time, however, I was right in my decision. Ray's OCD remained quiet and showed no signs of coming back to life in its new Zoloft-free environment. Whatever the Zoloft had been doing in Ray's brain, it wasn't holding back his OCD.

Ray has now been off of medication for several years. During that time his OCD has had minor flares but has never come close to regaining its former self. The only time he even thought about restarting a medication was during a stressful time when he was feeling both anxious and depressed. For about a month during a summer vacation from college, he was experiencing a myriad of negative symptoms: Sadness, irritability, lack of focus, trouble sleeping, general worrying, and poor self esteem. In all this, I couldn't clearly see OCD's hand, except for a time when he seemed unusually focused on his sleep and would say things like," I will never get anywhere because of my sleep problems. All I have worked for will be gone because I can't sleep." He would also ask me if I thought that his sleep problems would go away; that is, he sounded vaguely like he was asking for reassurance. It was during this time when Ray wondered if a medication would help him to feel better. I didn't stand in his way even though I suspected that with time and perspective these feelings would pass without the aid of any medication. I even called for a psychiatry appointment, but before Ray was seen (about one month after making the call), he was doing better and had decided not to restart any medication. During that month, Ray learned that negative feelings often pass if given enough time.

Ray's thoughts regarding his medication experience are similar to mine in that he feels that his ERP therapy was more important in helping him get over his OCD.

ΔΔΔΔ

For me, medication was a double edged sword. Medication has many uses, and for some, it may be the only thing they need to help them get over OCD, but that was not how it worked out for me. The experience that I have had with medication is like a love and hate relationship. I think my medication may have catalyzed me into do-

ing my therapy, but at the same time, I had to deal with side effects.

When my mom and I began to seriously approach my OCD, we first went to a psychiatrist for advice. The psychiatrist I saw offered no real therapeutic help but did suggest that I begin medication to see if it would help my symptoms. He wrote me a prescription for Prozac, and I took it for several months, gradually increasing my dose. I still remained anxious, and my OCD was still very much alive so it was decided that I should try another medication (Zoloft) to see if that would help me more. I don't think the Zoloft helped me anymore than the Prozac, but one thing I think the medications did help me with was that they dulled my anxiety enough so that I could face my therapy.

When we got to a point where my OCD had been fought back with ERP, we decided to wean me off of my medication that I was currently on (Zoloft). This proved to be a feat that would take months because even a small reduction in medication for me yielded drastic side effects. After dropping only a small amount on my dosage, I would have about a week's worth of nausea, weakness, and incredible irritability. Sometimes, I would even get this prickling sensation in my throat that made each second unbearable. From that experience, we learned that in order for me to get off the medication, we would have to go slow and steady.

Would I suggest taking medication? This question is one that depends highly on how someone personally responds to medicine and also on how severe their OCD symptoms are. If someone's OCD is to a point where they cannot go a minute without thinking about some sort of obsession (at one time, I was at this point), then medication is one of the tools that can be used. However, I personally believe that when OCD is more manageable and one's day-to-day life is not too consumed by OCD, then medication may not be the way to go. Also, ERP can give someone with OCD an additional tool to use by which to fight back any future emergence of obsessive thoughts.

ΔΔΔΔ

After my first visit with a psychiatrist, I started taking Zoloft and stayed on it for a couple of years. My experience with Zoloft was positive, and I know that it helped heal my brain from the stress that OCD had caused both me and Ray. But after taking it for awhile, I decided to try living without it. Even though I enjoyed the feelings the medication had provided for me, there was something about taking it that didn't feel right. I couldn't overcome my thinking that the real me no longer existed and had been replaced by a medication-spawned imposter. I knew this thinking wasn't entirely accurate. After all, I had been helped by Zoloft. If anything, the medication might have allowed me to have a more authentic life because it helped quell all the fear-induced thinking and the anxiety-ridden behavior that OCD had caused over so many years. I probably would have dismissed my concerns about the life Zoloft had helped me build if it hadn't been for one observation: I wasn't alone. My thinking on this wasn't unique; several writers, who have penned their experiences with mental illness, also have worried about what their medications were doing to their real selves and how by taking the pills, it clouded their sense of personal reality. Another book, written by a psychiatrist, spent hundreds of pages discussing what medications mean to those who take them and how for many, their pills allow them to feel "better than well." Even though such feelings are positive, some question their authenticity and wonder if it might not be better to try achieving those good feelings without the aid of medication.

Why many of us who take these medications feel conflicted about it isn't entirely clear to me. We feel good, so why can't we just sit back and enjoy the life our medications have helped form for us? I have no good answers to this dilemma and no advice for those who are struggling with their own questions. I did feel strongly, however, that I wanted to see if my new life that had been partially built by Zoloft could be maintained without it. Maybe Zoloft had helped rebuild my broken brain circuits to the extent that it was now possible to function without it.

After watching Ray's difficulty in weaning from Zoloft, I decided to bring myself down slowly and finally completed it after six months. With each step down, I felt a small jolt, like I had tripped while walking down some stairs and was in danger of falling the rest of the way down. But each time, I regained my equilibrium and returned to a baseline of happiness. Sometimes this return was quicker than others, but I always found my way back. At present, I have been medication free for several years and overall, am still happy with my decision. There have been times, however, when I feel the tug of depression and anxiety and wonder if my decision to stop Zoloft was wise. But by using the skills I learned while helping Ray, I haven't yet fallen too far and have found ways to stay healthy. Maybe the day will come when I need to restart my medication, and I'm prepared to do it. Why fight so hard and live a miserable life, when there's help? I'm just not there yet.

One additional thought about my medication experience: I have often wondered how effective I would have been in directing Ray's ERP therapy if I had been on Zoloft during the time we were undergoing his sessions. When I took Zoloft, I felt happy and often accepted the negative feelings that came my way. I felt those feelings, but I didn't worry about what those feelings were telling me. Was it possible that had I been on Zoloft during the worst of Ray's OCD that I might not have fought it so hard? Instead, maybe I would have thought, "Oh well, this is what life has given me, so I guess I will have to accept it and go on my way." Maybe I wouldn't have had the intensity that I often used to keep fighting Ray's OCD. Whenever I think about this, I'm reminded of a story about a woman who decided to get divorced after she had stopped her medication for depression. Her doctor wondered about this decision and suggested that she should go back on her medication, but she refused. She had realized that her medication had resulted in her accepting a bad situation and now that she was off of it, she was ready to move on and get out of her bad marriage. In this situation, it was her medication that had stalled her progress. Maybe my medication would also have stalled our progress in dealing with Ray's OCD. Anyway, it's something to think about.

Medications for OCD: Additional ideas

Instead of serving a life-saving role for Ray, his medications were more like a crutch that he used for support until he healed. What saved him was the ERP therapy and after that therapy had worked its magic, Ray no longer needed his crutch and put it away, hoping that he would never need it again. But, we keep it in the back of the closet and are prepared to dig it out, dust it off, and put it to use if the time ever comes when Ray needs it again.

If anyone would ask me advice on whether they or their loved ones should take medications for OCD, my answer would be simply: Maybe. Knowing that this answer is about as useless as using a spoon to dig a large hole, it's still the best one I have. I can't resolve it any better; there is still too much that is unknown about how the medications work and why individuals respond so differently to the same medication. Until the time comes that research can give us definitive answers about the role of medications in treating OCD, the best we can do is to ask endless questions, talk to each other about our experiences, and use ourselves as guinea pigs in our own personal experiments. But, I would also add this: Be careful who you listen to. Because science has yet to clearly state what these medications do and how they are to be used, opinion is often given more weight than it should. And, these opinions are frequently given with such force and certainty that we can easily mistake them for fact.

There are several books that have been written whose author's sole thesis was to discredit psychiatric medications. These authors make several claims: No studies have ever proven that the medications work, pharmaceutical companies are pushing ineffective medications because of the desire for large profits, and psychiatrists are often paid by the medication's makers to push the pills onto their patients. Some of these books are so well referenced and professionally written that I worry that they have convinced many of their readers that medications have no role in the treatment of mental disorders. This isn't true, of course; many lives have been saved because these medications were available, and I think it's a huge disservice to those who are suffering from mental disorders to be bombarded with such confusing information. What these authors have done is simply to cherry pick the studies they cite. In other words, they reference only that information which supports their ideas and ignore those studies that claim otherwise. They don't tell the whole story but only a portion of it. It's like someone who only allows us to see the upper portion of a landscape and not the whole picture. If we can only see the sky portion of that picture, then we would be fooled into thinking that we are looking at a representation of a sky and miss the other elements in that picture (ie, trees, rivers, flowers, rocks). Of course, these authors wouldn't dare write their books that disparage the use of psychiatric medicines if there existed good, definitive studies that clearly showed how people benefit from taking these medications.

For many of us, we have an additional source of confusion when it comes to deciding about using medications to treat a mental disorder: Our families. If we're lucky, our families are supportive. They ask the professionals questions, read every available source, discuss various options, and once a decision is made, stand quietly by until their support is needed again. And if a decision turns out wrong, they don't assign blame or tell us how stupid we were but dig in once again to help us find another plan that might work. But, I suspect that many of us who have OCD aren't as lucky and face family members who question our decisions regarding medications, especially if those decisions involve children. I once heard from a family member after Ray had been taking an SSRI for several months, "Do you really know what that medication is doing to his brain?" Here I was trying to rescue my son from OCD and at the same time was having to defend my decisions. I certainly didn't need the extra doubt that maybe I was doing something as bad as damaging my child's brain. I'm embarrassed to admit that I let that comment get to me and because of it, I spent hours needlessly worrying. What I should have done instead was to tell that family member to bug off or say something like, "If you're not going to help us get through this challenge, will you at least get the hell out of the way?"

Another idea about medications that's worth thinking about: Just because medications are started it doesn't mean that they will always be needed. When I finally got around to asking Ray's psychiatrist about the chances that Ray could successfully come off his Zoloft, he told us that it was about 50-50. But, he also said that since Ray had responded well to the ERP therapy that Ray's chances were probably better. This made sense. Ray had worked so hard during therapy that it was likely that he had built up some healthy brain circuits to counteract his defective OCD ones. In other words, his therapy had changed his brain and in doing so, had lessened his OCD. And, with his OCD under better control via his new brain pathways, he would no longer need any medication.

There is one positive idea about having a mental disorder that often gets lost in all the negative symptoms, the dysfunction, and the devastation: We have the power to change our brains and in doing so, can gain some control of our mental disorders. This doesn't happen as clearly with physical conditions. No amount of cognitive therapy will ever spark a diabetic's pancreas to start making insulin again or cause a tumor to suddenly start shrinking. Of course, therapy can help someone deal with the fear, pain, and loss of freedom that often occurs with these types of physical conditions. A cancer patient who has a positive outlook, for example, will be more likely to follow through with treatment, take better care of themselves, and stay engaged with the world. But, therapy can't directly affect the causes of physical disorders like it can with mental ones, such as depression and OCD. In mental disorders, therapy can alter the very structures that are causing the trouble. This happens because circuits in our brain can form and change in amazing ways. The same brain functions that we use every day to learn, solve new problems, and generate new ideas are the very ones that can also be used to heal ourselves from mental disorders. It's like using the tools we already have to build something fantastic, but we first have to learn new and different ways of using those tools.

Stopping Enabling

The severity of someone's OCD is affected by the choices they make. Some of what they do causes their OCD to worsen, but other actions can make it less painful. This isn't unique to mental disorders, like OCD, but is common to all illnesses. Diabetics fare much better, for example, when they actively check their blood sugars or carefully decide what foods to eat. Those who have OCD, however, also need to guard against those activities that feel helpful but are only serving to eventually worsen their OCD, like a smoker who enjoys his nicotine rush but increases his chance of lung cancer every time he lights up. With OCD, there are many choices that can be made and learning how to manage those choices is an important part of dealing with OCD.

Like many of his fellow sufferers of OCD, Ray tried to avoid anything that triggered his obsessions. His thinking was that since he was already so stressed with his OCD that he should avoid whatever it was that made his obsessions worse. It makes sense that he would think this; after all, when we sprain our ankle do we try to run on it or do we keep our weight off it until it heals? Any sensible person would wait, rest their ankle, take some tentative steps after the pain lessens, and when most of the pain has improved, start walking again. With OCD, however, this pain avoidance doesn't help with healing, but instead, paradoxically makes a person's life worse. Once someone who has OCD starts actively avoiding their triggers, it becomes very difficult to stop, like trying to stop an avalanche after it gets going. In time, the list of triggers can grow so large that it actually becomes easier to stop trying to live at all. For some who have OCD, their lives can become so constrained that they no longer leave their homes, eat their food, allow themselves to be touched by others, or even to talk to other people. In the attempt to avoid their fears, they have lost their lives. In the beginning, I helped Ray avoid his triggers. Seemingly harmless

238

acts, such as carrying extra hand sanitizer, making an unscheduled bathroom stop, or opening a door, eventually caused Ray to become less willing to fight his OCD. Why fight the anxiety when he had my help avoiding it? These actions were so small that I didn't realize that they were forming a bad habit for Ray, and I wasn't aware of the dangers they presented. Bad habits take time to form; smokers and drug addicts don't become addicted after smoking a handful of cigarettes or taking a few hits of a drug, and those with OCD who avoid their triggers don't appear to be adversely affected the first few times it happens. But in time, these imperceptibly small acts can build into a new way of behaving that is entirely dictated by the whims of OCD. In fact, if given enough time and leeway, OCD can hijack entire lives, telling someone where to go, who to talk to, what jobs are acceptable, and how to spend their free time.

For many, it's counterintuitive to think that helping someone who has OCD avoid their triggers would be wrong. Aren't we, especially parents, supposed to help alleviate the pain and anxiety in those we love? If we can, shouldn't we keep our loved ones far away from what they fear and what causes them so much anguish? It feels cruel and inhumane to force our loved ones to repeatedly face what they fear, but that is exactly what we need to do if they are to have a chance for an OCD-free life. Helping them avoid what they fear only tells their OCD that it can demand more, and inevitably, it will. OCD's first demands are often simple, asking that a door be opened, for example, or for a certain path to be avoided, but in time, it will ask for more until eventually, it may refuse to let someone leave their home or have a lasting relationship. As hard as it is, it's necessary for those of us who have loved ones with OCD to never validate it by listening to its demands. Instead, we need to listen carefully to what our loved ones tell us and to decide who is really making the request. If it's OCD in charge, then we need to stand firm, secure in the knowledge that our refusals to comply will help keep our loved one's OCD in check.

Helping someone who has OCD avoid their triggers is just one way in which OCD often tricks us into doing its bidding. The other main way is to involve us in the performing of compulsions, the behaviors that someone with OCD performs in an attempt to alleviate their anxiety. Compulsions come in many sizes and flavors, from simple (eg, confessing bad thoughts) to amazingly complex (eg, performing multi-step rituals) and from commonly-used ones (eg, hand washing) to unique variations. The involvement of loved ones in compulsions can be remote and indirect, such as repeatedly buying hand sanitizer or washing endless loads of laundry, or our involvement can be more complicated, such as washing our own hands when we don't think it's necessary or changing our clothes when it's requested of us. If we're not careful, our own lives can be commandeered by OCD until we become its puppets, not moving until OCD pulls a string.

Before I caught onto OCD's tricks, I had unknowingly let myself get sucked into helping Ray with his compulsions. I had bought gallons of hand sanitizer, washed loads of laundry, and had changed more sheets than many housekeepers who work at a hotel. I had also become his own personal doorman by opening every door for him, his priest by listening to his endless confessions, and his valet by doing almost everything he requested of me. By the time I finally realized the damage my complicity was causing, I had already spent countless hours and tremendous energy listening to Ray's OCD and doing what it requested. And, even after I knew that I had to stop helping Ray with his compulsions there was still one large problem that had to be solved. How do I stop? Ray had gotten so used to me being involved that to immediately stop would probably cause him more harm than good, like I was suddenly taking away his life-support system before he had healed enough to breathe on his own. The only option that I could think of at this point was to gradually extricate myself from

Ray's OCD by refusing to do some of the simpler requests, such as not opening certain doors or not responding to some of his confessions. To ease Ray into dealing with the new me, I first explained to him that it was best if I no longer honored OCD's requests. I also told him that each time we performed yet another compulsion, we were taking a step away from where we needed to be (ie, mentally healthy). Finally, I told him that it wasn't out of meanness or hatred that I decided to no longer help him but out of a strong desire to do what was best for him.

Ray hated my newly-discovered method of helping him. Where before he could count on me to do whatever was asked, I now balked at even the simplest requests. I no longer blindly followed his instructions, but instead, would hesitate, point out how much I hated participating in his compulsions, and remind him that each day, I would do less. Ray often reacted like I was hurting him; he yelled at me, threatened to hurt himself by not doing his homework, stomped away from me, and refused to interact further with me. Many times, I was tempted to revert back to our old ways, just to save time, energy, and mental strength, but I also knew that if Ray was to get better, we needed to dig in, hold tight, and weather whatever storm OCD threw against us.

As committed as I was to not complying with OCD's requests, I was sometimes forced to give in and go along. OCD is relentless in how it tortures its sufferers, and there were times when it was obvious that Ray couldn't take much more. And at such moments, I didn't have the heart to add to his misery. Even during these times, however, I wouldn't just blindly comply but would often justify my actions by saying such things as, "You know it's not a good idea for me to open this door for you because it's what your OCD wants, but I know that you have a test tomorrow and need to study, so I will help you this time, but I might not the next time you ask." Or, "You understand that it's not right for me to reassure you every time you tell me that you have a bad thought, but for now, I will tell you that you are a good person and don't need to confess your thoughts to me. But, if you ask me again within the next hour, I will pretend that I didn't hear." With these words, Ray got some relief but knew that it wouldn't always be forthcoming.

With time, persistence, a lot of explaining, and some yelling, I was finally a nonparticipant in Ray's compulsions. Even today, he sometimes forgets and tries to engage me in a compulsion-like behavior, mostly those that are related for his need of reassurance. Sometimes, we aren't immediately aware that Ray is asking for reassurance, but we usually catch on after the third or fourth request. At these times, I usually say something like," You know Ray, that is the fourth time you asked what would happen if you flunk some test, don't you think that maybe this idea is caught up in some of your OCD pathways and maybe we should just let it be." And on the rare occasion when he persists, I revert to my OCD-busting ways and tell him, "Now, I know this is OCD. Do not ask me again. I will not answer."

One of my many regrets I have with regards to Ray's OCD was that it took so long for me to realize how my actions were hurting him. I have often wondered if his OCD would have reached the severity it did if I hadn't been so accommodating to it and had not let it get so comfortable in our lives. But, we will never know. My advice to anyone who is facing down their own OCD monster is to be very careful in how you treat it. If you give it an inch, it will try to take a mile; know that you when you validate it in any way it will only feed off that validation and get larger. And the bigger it becomes, the harder it is to evict from your lives.

Even though Ray couldn't understand why accommodating his OCD wasn't good for him at the time when his OCD was at its worst, he now gets it.

ΔΔΔΔ

Any mental health professional will tell you that doing your compulsions only worsens your OCD. Even though intuitively this doesn't make sense (it often feels a little better after doing a compulsion), it is important to understand this principle because if OCD is to be beaten, it is necessary for anyone who has OCD to stop doing compulsions.

Logically, going through with compulsions is counterproductive. For anyone to get over OCD, they have to learn that their thoughts are not real but are only a product of OCD. By continuing with compulsions, someone with OCD is giving more into the misconception that the thoughts are real and that they do merit some sort of compulsion. For example, during my OCD, I asked my mom to wash my blankets and clothes all the time because I had obsessions that these items were contaminated. She would do it, out of kindness, but the more she gave in to my requests, the worse my symptoms became. Within a short time, I insisted that she wash these items more frequently. The main reason these compulsions got worse is because my mom enabled them and because of this cycle, I had positively reinforced the idea that my thoughts were real. The thoughts were not challenged, and thus, they remained at the status quo.

When my mom started challenging my OCD and stopped enabling my compulsions, my OCD immediately threw out counterattacks. The first thing she started to do was to stop telling me my thoughts were okay and that I was not a horrible person. I frequently had thoughts that orbited around the idea that I was an unethical and deplorable human being because I had some thought that could be remotely interpreted as sexual. I would go straight to my mom and ask her to reassure me that I was not evil. When my mom stopped doing this, I plunged into anxiety because there was no longer some outside source that reminded me of my sanity and goodness. Then, my mom started refusing to participate in other compulsions, such as buying me hand sanitizer, washing my clothes, and even letting me wash my hands. The whole justification behind her actions was that my thoughts were nothing more than an illusion. Through her refusal to help me engage in my compulsions, my OCD was challenged, and I truly began to get the idea that my thoughts were not real and that they were only hurting me.

My OCD frequently fought back against my mom. Since her reassurance and enabling behavior (like letting me wash my hands or washing my clothes) was the only outlet through which I knew how to release my anxiety, that anxiety got pent up inside me and turned into rage. I can remember slamming doors, hitting at the walls in my house, and locking myself in my room for long periods of time. Sometimes, I got so angry at my mom that I wanted nothing more than to leave our house for good and find someone who would truly understand how bad my obsessions made me feel. But in the end, after I had undergone my therapy and realized how useless my compulsions were, I knew that she was right to stop enabling my OCD.

Managing Stress

Once Ray's OCD had been beaten back, and he was in control of his life, we switched out of OCD-fighting mode and into one of prevention. We now had confidence that if his OCD fires were ever to rage out of control again, we had the skills (ie, ERP therapy) to beat it back into submission. But, we also had learned how much that effort costs and decided that if there was any way to prevent Ray's OCD from ever regaining its strength, we needed to find it. It's like investing in simple equipment, such as smoke detectors and hand held fire extinguishers, that can be used to stop a small fire before it grows into something that needs an entire fire department. Many books on OCD suggest that one of the most important things that someone can do to help keep their OCD at bay is to manage their stress.

Events, such as marriages, divorces, births, and deaths, are times of immense stress, so it's not surprising that during these times, OCD takes advantage and digs in. But it can also worsen, and do so dramatically, during less intense times, such as moving away to college, transitioning between jobs, or even during downtimes, such as school breaks or family vacations. Several authors of OCD memoirs describe how their OCD got markedly worse when they went to college or when they got their first job. Sadly, during those times in their lives when they should have been excited and moving forward they were stopped by OCD. What Ray and I decided to do first in this area of stress management was to see if we could actively manage his environment and keep as much stress out of his life as we could. By doing this, we hoped to improve his odds of staying OCD free.

Knowing that we couldn't predict when the big, bad, and ugly things might happen to us, we focused on managing the smaller stresses of life. When Ray's OCD was at its worst, we didn't have the time or energy to worry about the little things, but now that he was once again among the mentally sound, we turned our attention to helping him manage his everyday stress. The first area we worked on was to improve his overall organization. Ray had never been one who kept good track of his things, such as cell phones, wallets, or homework papers. On most school days, we wasted large amounts of time looking for needed items and would often not find all of them, which would then cause a subsequent round of problems. To help alleviate this problem, I started a routine where I would look through his school bag, throw away any garbage that had collected, locate any papers that looked important, and remove any old papers from between the pages of his textbooks and place them in a folder. This took effort, and Ray was often unhappy with my school-bag interventions. But, it helped him keep track of those important items he needed. I also questioned him (endlessly, if you ask Ray) about what homework was due the next day, what projects were due within the week, and why he didn't get better grades on certain assignments. To help me, I took advantage of a computer system that his school had implemented by which parents could check on their kid's grades, attendance records, and disciplinary actions. Every day, I would check up on Ray and see if he was following through with his assignments. I know he got sick of me and my questions, but it helped keep his stress in check and improved his grades.

There were other, more unconventional, ways that we minimized Ray's stresses. Many parents would disagree with me on this, but I often gave Ray money so he could have fun. When many of his friends were being told to get a job if they wanted the extras in life, I just gave Ray the money. I didn't see the benefit of adding the stress of a job so that he could enjoy seeing movies with friends, eating out, or buying small items. I worried that it would be detrimental to his continued recovery from OCD if we had followed the well worn path that many parents use and force him to work at some low paying job just so he could learn the value of hard work and money. I figured that he would eventually learn that lesson, maybe just later than other kids his age.

Ray also found ways to keep his stress levels low, sometimes even in spite of my ideas. The best example of this was when he decided not to take driver's education at his school. We had talked about it; he had initially agreed; and I had contacted the teacher in charge, but when he requested that Ray come to his office and sign up, Ray never managed to find the time. Even after I questioned Ray about it and told him that it was a good idea for him to get his license with his classmates, he still found ways to "forget" signing up until it was too late. Ray finally admitted to me that he didn't want to deal with driver's education in addition to his other schoolwork. Another reason was that this class would require Ray to give up his PE class, the one time during his day that he felt relaxed. Once I understood Ray's thinking on this, I stopped pushing him to take driver's education. But, I also wondered if his decision might cause problems elsewhere for him. If he were the only one in his class not to have a license, would that cause him some embarrassment and maybe result in him being teased by his classmates? To prevent this, we devised a plan. If anyone gave him a hard time about not driving he was to tell them that his mother had made him an offer he couldn't refuse: He was to receive all the money that would have been spent on his car insurance. It worked; none of his classmates bothered Ray for not driving, especially after being told about his small fortune. (In total, Ray received about $2,000, the majority of which, he let me invest for him.)

Even though our goal was to minimize Ray's stress in life, we knew that it wasn't possible, or even desirable, to eliminate all stress. In fact, certain stresses are good for us and help us accomplish goals that we might not otherwise. Studying for tests or completing projects at work are areas where stress is present and can help us achieve our goals. Also, since stress is so prevalent in our lives, I knew that it

247

was important for Ray to learn how to handle it and remain resilient. Even though it was tempting to let Ray sit back and enjoy life, we both knew that that wasn't a good option. For Ray to succeed, he would have to face problems, deal with stress, handle failure, and do all of it without letting OCD gain a footing. But, how to find the balance? How to walk that delicate line between having enough good stress to foster healthy growth but not too much of the bad kind that hinders progress or allows OCD to grow? Much to my relief, Ray solved this problem on his own and found ways to increase the kind of stress that is helpful.

One of Ray's strong points is that he is competitive, and when he saw that some of his friends were taking the harder classes in school, he decided that he wouldn't sit back and let them get academically ahead of him. The problem, however, was that some of his teachers didn't think he could handle the tougher schedule and were hesitant to give him the required permission. I can understand why they thought this. For most of Ray's freshmen and sophomore years, his mind had been too occupied handling his OCD and not focusing on his classes. Even with this handicap, though, Ray did OK and got A's and B's in his classes, but it wasn't easy and at times, he struggled to get his work done. Because of this struggle, Ray's teachers didn't see his academic potential and thought it was best to keep him in the regular classes and not have him try the more challenging ones. Their attitude towards Ray actually made him angry and sparked something in him that I still don't understand.

To get past his teacher's roadblocks, Ray used several strategies. Sometimes, he simply insisted that he was going to take their classes regardless of their hesitations. To accomplish this, I had to sign a paper stating that I understood the situation and the teacher's viewpoint but would still allow Ray to take the class. In other words, if he failed, it wasn't the school's fault but mine. For one class, however, it wasn't so easy. Ray wanted to take a higher level math class but had not done well enough on a prerequisite test that all the students had taken. He had come close to doing well enough but was still several points away from the cutoff. Most students would probably have accepted the situation and decide to take the lower level class but not Ray. To get into the class he wanted, he took an online math tutorial over his summer break. Because he wanted to keep up with his friends, he spent his summer working on the tutorial, passed the necessary tests, and was allowed entry into the higher class.

Throughout high school, Ray was juggling two major stressors: Hard classes (good stress) and OCD (bad stress). There were times when he stumbled, wanted to quit, and regretted his decisions. I stood by and did what I could, helping him with assignments, keeping him organized, and encouraging him to hang on when he wanted to let go. I have always admired him for his persistence and for his stubbornness not to be left behind. He took on more than most students his age dared to and came out stronger and more confident. After seeing how he handled himself throughout his high school career, I knew that Ray wouldn't let the stresses of life stop him and would use his competitive spirit to spur him on.

Ray's competitiveness served him well and allowed him to overcome some of the deficits OCD had created. Many times, I wondered what I would have done if Ray hadn't possessed this characteristic. Would we have found other ways to foster good stress in his life so that he learned how to handle it or would we have kept all stress away from him because we feared that his OCD might strengthen if we didn't? We were lucky in this respect, which makes me wonder how others achieve the balance between having enough stress to keep moving forward but not too much where it causes problems. And, if anyone would ask my advice in how to help someone walk this delicate line, I would be hard pressed to give any solid ideas. I would, however, emphasize that it's important to find healthy challenges and to never just sit on the sidelines in life. It might take time and a lot of digging to find those challenges, but the return on that investment would be priceless.

Ray also realizes that stress has had different effects on his OCD depending on what type of stress he is experiencing and on what stage his OCD is in.

ΔΔΔΔ

In my experience, stress can help but also can make OCD worse. There have been several times when I can attribute stress to actually dimming my OCD symptoms, but there were also times when stress provoked my obsessions.

One example of how stress can actually help OCD happened recently during a summer vacation from college. During this vacation, I started to obsess about the possibility of not getting enough sleep because of insomnia. I worried that because of this sleep deficit, I would never achieve anything worthy. The interesting thing is that these thoughts became a problem because I was no longer taking classes. After school was over, my time was suddenly unstructured, and I was free to do and think about whatever I wanted. In other words, I had no stress because there were no expectations on me but that resulted in me focusing on OCD rather than on something productive. As soon as I found a new routine to follow, my obsessions quickly dissipated and my worrying ceased.

One important lesson I learned about myself is that if I have too much unstructured time, my OCD tries to get a foothold. Therefore, I have learned to always keep myself busy, active and never just sit at home without anything to do. I have learned that one way to keep OCD at bay is to plan out each day and to keep myself busy.

However, certain types of stress can be bad for OCD. Recently, for example, my OCD sometimes zones in on my grades. College classes are stressful, and the tests I have to study for and take are often very difficult. If I am uncertain as to how I did on a test, I can sometimes sense my OCD starting up. I will ruminate, continuously check online grading systems, and sometimes, even email my teacher to find out how I did. This kind of stress is not good because it can trigger my OCD.

One way in which I have found to help lessen the bad stress in my life is to keep organized. If my room is messy, for example, I often have a hard time dealing with the chaos, and my OCD might try to flare up. If I can't find my wallet, my cell phone, or my class notebook, I get stressed and end up wasting a lot of time. Therefore, it is imperative for me to keep my room, my papers, and my life organized.

Stress that results in the building up of self esteem or in the development of some kind of skill is good for many reasons and may even result in keeping OCD away. The stress that serves only to overwhelm, however, needs to be avoided at all costs because such stress makes it harder to fight back against OCD.

Exercise

Of all the OCD-managing ideas that we tried, exercise was the easiest for us to manage. All we had to do with this intervention is find ways to move. There weren't any specific techniques to master, like in ERP therapy, or any difficult balancing acts to perform, like in managing stress. We just had to get up and move. In fact, Ray had turned to physical activity as a way to help him deal with his OCD even before we considered using it in a more systematic form. Many times, when he was feeling the intensity of OCD we would venture to a nearby state park and go hiking or would walk along the river on our own property. Ray had learned that walking could help calm the turbulence of his OCD and allow him to feel more peaceful.

Even though there aren't many studies that directly link physical activity to improved OCD symptoms, there are a large number that describe how exercise improves other mental conditions, such as depression and decreased memory. Thanks to the sacrifice of countless rats and mice, who have been run on exercise wheels, placed in mazes to see how they can solve problems, and given up their brains to be sliced, diced, and examined, we know that exercise, at least in rodents, physically and chemically changes the brain in ways that are beneficial. It has been shown, for example, that exercise results in the birth of new neurons (brain cells) in the area of the brain responsible for memory (the hippocampus) and that the brains of elderly mice react differently (eg, express different genes) after exercise than those of younger ones.

Studies in humans, of course, can't be as controlled as those in rodents, but there still exists a lot of information that points to the benefits of exercise. It has been shown, for example, that among the elderly, those who had walked a lot had larger hippocampi and higher levels of an important brain substance (brain derived neurotrophic factor (BDNF)) than those who were more sedentary. College students also have improved memories and increased levels of BDNF after exercising. With regards to mental illness, the condition that has been studied the most with regards to exercise is depression. To date, many studies have shown that exercise can improve the symptoms of depression. In fact, some patients have even been able to push their depression into remission after adding exercise to their treatment regimen.

With all this information (and more being added each week) about the mental benefits of exercise, it seemed obvious that we should give it a try. Maybe by adding exercise to our daily routine we could improve Ray's chances of staying OCD free and mine of remaining depression free. Of course, we didn't think that exercise alone would either treat OCD or keep it at bay, but we wondered if it could help protect Ray's brain from additional OCD onslaughts. This idea was also fostered by the results of yet another study which showed that brain cells in rats that had been created because of exercise didn't respond to stress. In other words, an exercise-changed brain (at least in rats) was more buffered from the effects of stress than one whose owner had sat their way through life.

Ray led the way in this project by insisting we join a gym where he could do many different activities like lifting weights and running. I followed along and eventually, found a home among the treadmills where my endurance has gradually improved to the point where running is almost enjoyable. Throughout the last several years, our exercise experiment has undergone several modifications, such as changing gyms, buying our own equipment, trying different forms of exercise, and dealing with injuries, which forced both Ray and I to take prolonged breaks. One option we never took, however, was to give up, sit back down, and conclude that exercise has no role in our lives.

While we can't quantify the mental health benefits from our own exercise experiment, we have concluded one thing: Exercise helps. And, we have learned that the more we exercise the better we feel. Even though federal guidelines suggest that thirty minutes of moderate exercise about three times per week is enough to see health benefits, we found that much more than that was required for us to feel maximal mental health benefits. Not only did we need to exercise for more than three times each week, we also had to undergo intense exercise, such as running for several miles, using the elliptical machine, or biking using the higher resistance settings. For us to keep mentally healthy, we need to markedly raise our heart rates and to keep them there for a prolonged time. Currently, both Ray and I exercise almost daily and even try to keep up our routines while on vacation. It's become that important to us.

Exercise alone is not strong enough to keep the OCD woolies at bay. But, it helps. With exercise, I'm convinced that certain brain pathways bulk up and become stronger. And, when those pathways are needed to help deal with life's crises, they are fit, ready to go, and can fire when called upon. In a way, it's like exercise gives Ray's brain an added layer of protection against OCD. It might not be strong enough to repel an all out attack by OCD, but it can help turn back the repeated, smaller excursions that OCD often sends out.

Ray also thinks that exercise helps in maintaining his OCD-free life.

∆∆∆∆

During the worst times of my OCD, I often had nowhere to turn for comfort. People around me could not provide me relief because they were one of the sources of my OCD anxiety. Video games, movies, and food helped me through some of the tough times, but none of those activities provided me with a sense of self worth because after all, how much self improvement comes from those three things? It was not until my sophomore year of high school, in the midst of my OCD, that I stumbled upon fitness and began to realize the benefits it provided.

How often do you hear on the news and from doctors and mental health professionals about how good exercise is for you? Whether we exercise for our overall physical health or for our mental health, we all instinctually know that the healthier we are, the happier we are, and for those of us who have OCD, the sounder our minds. I found that exercise was one of the keys to getting over my OCD.

I first began exercising as a requirement for school. I was enrolled in a personal fitness class, and it was there that I learned the basics of weight training. After several months of basic weight training, I noticed significant changes in my physique that helped me feel good about myself. Where success in academics had provided me with a sense of self worth, the process of studying and trying to get good grades was too difficult and stressful. With bodybuilding, however, I had found something fun and exciting, and it provided me with a sense of self esteem that I had not felt in years.

Soon after I started seriously weight training, I began running. What I loved so much about running was the mental relief it provided me from my OCD thoughts. While I was running, I felt free in a sense that my mind was too preoccupied with the huffing and puffing that comes with running. The more I ran, the less I thought about OCD, and the greater relief it gave me from my anxieties. After running for five or six miles, my thoughts stayed at bay for awhile and allowed me a short time where my OCD wasn't in control.

Other Ideas

Even though Ray and I have gathered many tools to use against OCD, we continue to look for more. Our experience has taught us that OCD will never give up but will always try to come back and cause us trouble. We hope that when it does, the tools we already have and our skills in using them will suffice to destroy OCD, but we also suspect it will try new ways to return that could be immune to our methods. Because of this possibility, we are always on the lookout for new ideas that can be added to our OCD-busting arsenal.

One new method that Ray and I have just started working on is meditation and mindfulness. For several years, this topic has been included on the schedule at the annual OCD conference, an indication that the experts in OCD think it's a useful method. Even though no expert has said that meditation can replace the main therapy for OCD (ie, exposure and response prevention therapy (ERP)), they are suggesting that it can help deal with some of OCD's symptoms. This makes sense. When obsessions are out of control like a runaway truck, something as gentle and passive as meditation isn't going to do much. I know that when Ray was at his worst, I couldn't even get him to sit in one place for long, so I know that merely telling him to quiet his thoughts and meditate would have been futile. But, maybe meditation can keep mild OCD from getting worse or can help push back some remaining OCD symptoms after someone has undergone their ERP therapy. I also hope to use it as an OCD-prevention method for Ray.

Some would probably scoff at the idea that something as low key as meditation and mindfulness could help in the treatment of mental illness. It looks too much like sleep or is too entwined in the alternative medicine area to command much respect. But, researchers in neurobiology have looked into the effects of meditation and have discovered that it can actually change brain functions.

When the experts on meditation (namely monks) were placed in a brain scanner and their brains were imaged, it became clear that meditation can significantly alter a person's brain. Not surprisingly, the observed changes were in brain areas that can affect a person's outlook in life. The clearest example of this is that the brains of meditators have more function in the left side of their frontal lobes when compared to their right sides. This is important because the left side is known to control positive emotions and the more it functions, the more positive someone is likely to be. With the results of these types of studies, it's easier to accept the idea that meditation can be a powerful ally in the treatment of mental illnesses.

Ray looked into using meditation and mindfulness to help him with OCD during his latest episode and had realized its potential. Even though he didn't pursue it as thoroughly as he could have, he thought it helped him deal with the anxiety his OCD caused and has promised me that he will continue reading about meditation and learning about it. I also remind him about this method whenever he mentions to me that he still has lingering symptoms from this latest OCD flare. His symptoms are currently so mild that a gentle method like meditation could probably help him get the rest of the way to an OCD-free state.

When we first heard of meditation and mindfulness, we dismissed it because it looked too complicated. We were busy and didn't want to make the effort to learn about it. But in time, we have discovered how wrong that thinking was. Learning to do meditation is not hard at all. Of all the ideas we have learned about meditation, the one that has stayed with us the most is simply this: There is no wrong way to do meditation. One doesn't have to hire a Tibetan monk or travel to some mountain retreat and stay there for a month to learn effective meditation. All anyone has to do is to learn some basics, such as sitting still, closing one's eyes, taking some deep breaths, and refocusing one's thoughts. These simple actions, of course, aren't enough to make someone an expert in meditation, but they are a way to get started and even, to begin feeling some positive effects.

There is one final idea on dealing with OCD that we would like to address. This idea doesn't require the obtaining of a skill like ERP or the alteration of one's habits like exercise or stress management but requires something more subtle. We also didn't use this idea nearly as much as we should and hope that others with OCD don't forget about it. It's simply this: Rest and relaxation. During the times when Ray's OCD was out of control, we pushed back against it for months on end. I was particularly stubborn about it and would often not let Ray off the hook about his OCD. I kept our focus on OCD and only rarely allowed us to take a break. Because of this approach, I let OCD take over our lives even more than what it already was.

Even with something as encompassing as OCD, it's still important to find ways to live a healthy life. There are movies to see, books to read, parties to attend, birthdays to celebrate, and friends to visit. Time and energy must be preserved for all these activities; otherwise, OCD will take even more. Of course, until OCD is effectively dealt with, it will come along for the ride and will probably even make some demands, but my advice is this: Let it. Find those activities where OCD can come and not cause too much trouble. Accommodations for OCD may have to be made, but go anyway. Show OCD that no matter how large, noisy, and smelly it becomes that the life it has invaded is still thriving and growing.

Here I would like to address the loved ones, especially the parents, of those who have OCD: Please take care of yourself. In fact, it's critical to your loved one's success in treating their OCD that you look after your own needs. One way that you can do this is by taking a day or two off every month from OCD and use it to do something fun, indulgent, and completely self-absorbing. And, you are to do this guilt free. You are not to think of your loved one during this time, worry about them, or to contact them. I realize that upon hearing these words, you might think something like, "But my daughter can't take a day off from OCD, so why should I? She can't have fun, so I don't feel right indulging in something fun." Or, you might be worried that if you aren't immediately available to your loved one that something bad will happen because of their OCD. I understand. But, you also need to remember that your loved one doesn't have a chance in beating back their OCD without you, and if you become burned out, exhausted, or sick, you can't help them any more. You are a critical part of their treatment and because of that, it's imperative that you stay strong. As the saying goes, "Retreat when you must, live to fight another day."

And finally, to our fellow sufferers of OCD: Please let your loved ones have some time to themselves. They have worked so hard in helping you deal with your OCD and have given up much of their life to get you through. They deserve this time. Even if you are frightened and want them to stay home, you need to let them go for a little while. They'll be back. In the meantime, find something to do. Maybe you could take a walk, read a book, watch a movie, or if all else fails, lie down on your bed and wait. But, be sure to smile (fake it if you have to) when your loved one is preparing to leave and reassure them that you will be OK until they get back. You need them to help you get over OCD, so please do what you can to help them stay strong.

Part V – Additional Issues on OCD

Aftermath of OCD

Once we felt confident that Ray's OCD was on the run, we celebrated. We laughed. We rested. We rehashed our war stories, embellishing them by emphasizing the more exciting elements and by adding in humor to help us cope with our memories. But soon, we realized that Ray had another problem to face down: The aftermath of OCD. We had expected that once OCD was essentially gone that all would be fine and that Ray would resume his life. He did, of course, but there was one realization that we hadn't expected. Ray was behind. For all the time he was mired in OCD, his classmates had been moving along in their lives, learning, experimenting, and developing relationships. Ray couldn't do any of these things when he was under OCD's control; it was all he could do to get through the day without melting down.

To help us describe what it's like to deal with the aftermath of OCD, we have often compared it to dealing with a tornado. When the tornado (ie, OCD) is on top of you, all you can think about is surviving. You hide in your basement and wait (or undergo treatment in the case of OCD), hoping that when it's over, you will still be alive. Other considerations don't even cross your mind; you just want to live. And, when the tornado has moved on and you realize that you've made it, you're amazed, thrilled, and relieved. You may notice that your house has been destroyed but that isn't too significant to you at the time. You just want to celebrate your survival. You might even crawl to the top of your destroyed house, sit down with a glass of wine, and give a toast to your incredible experience. But then, it slowly occurs to you that your house is gone, and all your possessions have been scattered. There is no choice but to rebuild, but where to start? You also get angry that you have to deal with this and feel jealous of your neighbors whose houses remain intact. Why didn't they have to deal with the tornado and its aftermath? And, why do they always look away when you meet them like there's something wrong with you? It wasn't our fault the damned tornado took out our house; they were lucky it didn't hit them. But in time, you make peace with your situation and start rebuilding. After all, there really isn't any other choice.

Not surprisingly, Ray quickly became depressed when he realized how far behind he had fallen because of his OCD. He didn't have many friends because he had been too busy wrestling with his obsessions; he hadn't participated in any extracurricular activities because he didn't have any energy left over after attending school; and his grades weren't as good as he had hoped because he couldn't tune out his obsessions and listen to what his teachers were saying. Even with me constantly reminding him of how much he had already accomplished by fighting back his OCD, he felt low. Some days, he didn't even want to try any more and thought about quitting altogether. But, he didn't. He kept plodding along and in time, regained his strength and enthusiasm.

Ray felt the worst when he compared the accomplishments of others to his own record. He saw that many of his fellow students had more awards, scholarships, and had been invited to attend more renowned universities. Even though he had just completed one of the most difficult journeys that anyone could ever take (ie, undergoing therapy to treat OCD), he didn't feel proud of that accomplishment. His work had been done in private where no one could watch. There are no trophies, medals, award dinners, media attention, or even, a simple congratulation that is presented to those who win their life back from OCD. What Ray and his fellow sufferers of OCD accomplish is more impressive than anything I have ever seen and yet, no one else witnesses it. If it were up to me, I would grant automatic entry into any university or institution, approve any proposal, and publish any article written by those who have fought back their OCD. These people impress me. Now, I just have to figure out how to convince the rest of the world.

Admittedly, there was a brief time when I was jealous of those students who were striving past Ray and doing wonderful things. But, all that has changed. Now, when I hear about some kid in our area who has won a certain award, broken a certain record, or been accepted to some elite college, I no longer feel jealous. I congratulate said kid and their parents and go on my way. Privately, I think, "If you want to see true success, you need to know about what Ray has done." What anyone has to do to heal from OCD is the most laudable act I can imagine. The obstacles overcome, the pain endured, and the distance covered is unimaginable to those who aren't forced to take this journey. I can tell you, honestly, that I no longer feel any admiration for the awards given to others. The true victory goes to people like Ray, who have faced their worst fears and have come out of it better and stronger.

Ray took some convincing, but he finally accepted the idea that his life wasn't over. Maybe certain doors had been closed to him (eg, certain prestigious universities or scholarships), but there was still so much he could do. With hard work, persistence, and time, I knew it was possible for him to catch up to his classmates and would probably, even surpass many of them. He just had to overcome the funk he was in, decide to try, and not worry about what would happen. As long as he was moving forward, going to classes, thinking about colleges, and attempting to reconnect with friends, I was confident that it would work out for Ray. And, it has. Today, he is in his second year of college and taking courses that many couldn't handle. He is looking ahead to a career in medicine or research and is actively making plans to get there. He also has friends whom he hangs out with on a regular basis. All this happened for him because he didn't give up. OCD may have knocked him down, but he found the strength to pick himself up, brush himself off, and start out again to live his life.

When dealing with the aftermath of something as destructive as OCD, one question inevitably arises: How much of this damage is permanent? In other words, can all the mess that OCD creates be cleaned up or will some of it remain with us for the rest of our lives? It's like dealing with some large disaster, such as a huge oil spill or a category five hurricane. You know that a lot of the damage will be cleaned up and rebuilt, but you aren't sure how much. And, even if you are successful in erasing the visible aspects of the disaster, like skimming off the surface oil from a spill, you still think about the less visible parts. How much oil is still there, under the surface, leaking into our water or food supply? Can we really be sure that it's no longer something to worry about?

For Ray, it's too early to tell how much OCD has permanently affected his life. We have rebuilt much of what OCD had destroyed during his earlier years. The main structures of his life, that is, his friends, family, and college are now standing strong again, and at first glance, Ray looks unaffected by his OCD experience. But, I suspect that there are elements to his life that have been scarred by OCD and in time, will make themselves known. Maybe he will be more hesitant in forming intimate relationships because of how OCD had affected him; maybe he will worry about taking on certain responsibilities because he remembers how OCD can take over; or perhaps he will decide not to take some risks because he thinks his luck won't hold out. After all, where was his luck when it came to parceling out those OCD genes? But, I'm not too worried about Ray. His OCD was caught and treated when he was still relatively young and before it had time to permanently alter all the important parts of his life. Also, I will never forget what OCD tried to do to Ray and will always be vigilant to any after effects it may try to exert. I'm not afraid to tell Ray when I think OCD is involved in his actions, regardless of how subtle or indirect the effect. Maybe this hypervigilance isn't necessary, but I am not willing to take the chance.

At this point in his life (age nineteen), Ray sees some after effects of his OCD, especially from his sexual obsessions. But, he is also committed to continuing his efforts to overcome all these residual problems.

ΔΔΔΔ

The biggest toll that OCD has taken on me is primarily my loss of both sexual relationships and long-term relationships with women. For a long time, OCD used sexuality as a way to torment me and made it so miserable that at one point, I could not even be in the presence of any female (even young children). Thus, I developed a sort of fear of women as well as a lacking of understanding in how to talk or be friends with them. Even to this day, I still struggle to get over this thinking and find ways to move on.

Many of my close friends are in relationships or have been in one at one time. They frequently ask me about why I do not have a girlfriend, and I often tell them that I don't have the time for such a relationship. But, the truth is I still hesitate to enter into such a relationship. Because of my sexual obsessions, I spent so much time and energy avoiding anything of a sexual nature that I essentially shut down that part of my life.

However, this is something I am not happy about. I know that in order to fully develop as a person, close emotional connections are necessary because through caring for others can you feel emotions such as passion, true love, and happiness. I do not want to live the rest of my life without feeling these emotions and dooming myself to a life lived in loneliness. I want someone I can spend the rest of my life with and love to be around. So, I am avidly working to get this part of my life back on track to the point where I can enjoy a long-term relationship and find solace in being with someone.

I constantly work to meet more people. My OCD took many opportunities from me to meet new people and prevent-

ed me from having the friends that I should have had. I also see it as my duty to get back at my OCD by making up for all that lost time and lost friendship. I hope that if I continue to meet new people, I can begin to love and appreciate them in a way that I never had the chance to do when struggling with OCD.

I plan to focus my energy on getting out into the world and meeting with, talking to, and learning about other people. I want to learn how to fully empathize with people and understand their points of view because only then, will I be able to build strong relationships. I hope that people who make me the happiest are women because then, I know that I will have gotten back all that OCD took from me.

∆∆∆∆

In me, OCD wasn't recognized for decades and because of that, my life has often taken OCD-directed paths. But even with OCD partially in control, I've done all right. I've limped along, making my way in this life as best I could. I got through medical school and pediatric residency and have practiced pediatrics in a rural area. All of this I somehow accomplished in spite of OCD and the burdens it forced me to carry. Many who have OCD are similar to me; we do well professionally and take on more responsibility than a lot of people. Even with the OCD monkey perpetually on our backs, we trudge forward, determined to make our contributions. However, many of our OCD brethren aren't so lucky and have been forced to live more compromised lives. Their OCD keeps them from holding jobs, forming families, maintaining friends, and in some cases, from even leaving their homes or eating.

Where I see OCD's effects the strongest in my life is in friendships, or in my case, the lack thereof. Because one of my obsessions was to worry about what others thought of me, I was anxious in social situations, and it showed. Many times, I simply did what many

267

do: I avoided those situations that would trigger my anxiety. I would either not go somewhere where I was expected to talk to others, or I would go and not talk. I'm sure that those around me thought I was either shy or arrogant. To make my situation even worse, there were times when I forced myself to talk, but because of my anxiety, I was awful. I would ramble, interrupt, nervously laugh, repeat myself, and generally, create an annoyance. How could anyone with these tendencies befriend others in a meaningful way? Perhaps if the right people had come along in my life or if I had received therapy, I could have created some lasting friendships, but as it happened, it took too many years for me to realize my problems and then, it was too late. To this day, I lack the skills to generate and maintain lasting friendships. My long-standing, unrecognized, and untreated OCD has kept me from having the kinds of friendships we all need.

Ray has also struggled with developing friendships because of what OCD has done to him, but unlike me, he has realized this early on and can now actively work on correcting this deficit.

ΔΔΔΔ

OCD took a lot from me in regards to talking to and emotionally connecting with people. When I struggled with OCD, every waking thought was directed towards avoiding contamination or avoiding sexual thoughts. I felt like I was fighting off leopards for my survival in the jungle. Each day, all I would feel is the stress that it must feel like during the midst of a war; I was honestly that anxious. I would ward off any person who I thought could trigger my OCD thoughts (especially girls) and would avoid making new friends out of fear that I might contaminate them.

I ignored people in my class in high school so that they would get a bad impression of me and stop trying to talk to me. I did this for

268

them and not because I was selfish or egocentric. I thought I was keeping them away from the evil that was in me and that if I let them into my life, I would only be exposing them to the contamination that my OCD said was my responsibility. Thus, I spent several years in high school cultivating my fears and not cultivating any social experiences. I ended up as an OCD-free junior in high school, but I was also a junior who had almost no social experience. I did not know how to make proper jokes, how to make people think I was intelligent or mature, or how to make really good friends. Because of my OCD, I have had to work hard to get myself to a point where I am not completely awkward or off-putting.

As of today, I am still not where I want to be socially. Over a recent Thanksgiving break, for example, I took a trip to Costa Rica with a class, and I tried as hard as I could to make friends with people in that group. I would take extra effort to hang out with them and think ahead about interesting topics to talk about. However, I just never quite had it; at least, not to where I wanted to be. After talking to them for a little while, I would get frustrated about how little I could think of to say and how quiet I would become after only ten minutes of talking. At times, I got so frustrated about my capabilities of conversation that I just gave up.

However, as I have realized, I am slowly getting better. I am now better able to get a friendly and interesting conversation going with my peers than I was a year ago. I have even found that I want to know more about people and find them inherently more interesting than I had just a little while ago. Recently, I went to a college party and found that I could talk to everyone there. I made funny jokes and came off as confident in a way I never dreamed I could have done just a short while ago. This progress has inspired me to keep talking to people no matter how frustrated I may get or how much I may want to give up.

ΔΔΔΔ

When we were actively fighting Ray's OCD, we didn't think about its aftermath. After all, when one's house is being torn apart by a tornado, there isn't time or energy to think about much other than surviving. But as I was running for safety and dragging Ray with me, I briefly wondered if there were things I could take with me and keep safe. As I quickly looked around, I saw many things I wanted to save (friendships, family relationships, career opportunities, financial security, hobbies) but doubted I could. They were either too heavy to move in such a short notice or were in a location where I couldn't get to them in time. So, we left most of them, hoping that they would miraculously remain intact but knowing that wasn't likely. Of all things that got left behind, however, there was one that worried me the most: Our relationships with those around us. I suspected that many of those relationships wouldn't survive, but I hoped that some would pull through. I also hoped that for those that were damaged, we would find ways to repair them and make them whole and functional once again. But, I also accepted the idea that none of our relationships would be left standing when we finally emerged from our OCD hell.

When it was all over and Ray was once again healthy, we looked around and took stock of what was left with regards to our relationships. We were dismayed, but not surprised, by what we found. Most of his friends were long gone. This had been expected; after all, teenagers don't know much about mental illness, and his friends couldn't understand what Ray was going through. They had moved on and had made other friends when it was obvious to them that something was wrong with Ray and when he couldn't engage with them like he had before. Fortunately, this situation has improved for Ray and now, he has friends that he often hangs out with. He sometimes wishes that he has more close friends and is working on developing those kinds of relationships. I'm not too worried about this aspect of Ray's life; he has made progress in this area and has a desire to continue getting better. And, where there is a desire to work for something, progress follows.

Our closest relationships fared better than those with Ray's friends but were still severely affected. I had hoped that these relationships would have been protected because they were more entrenched in our lives. They existed deeply in our inner sanctums where I thought they would be most buffeted from the OCD winds, but I learned quickly that I was wrong in this thinking. In many ways, it was these relationships that felt the full force of OCD. It was more like we were dealing with a tornado within our own home instead of one that was swirling outside its walls. We learned early on, that if these relationships were to have any chance of surviving, we would have to either tame the tornado (ie, get rid of the OCD) or enclose if off (ie, hide it) whenever we could. Of course, we would have liked to have had a third option: Not worrying at all because we had faith that our relationships were unbreakable and would be left intact no matter what OCD tried to do. But for us, this option wasn't available, and our choices were only two, either let the OCD destroy our relationships or wrestle it into those areas where its effects were less direct. We had hoped that if those around us could only hear the OCD tornado raging from behind closed doors and not feel its direct force, then maybe they would stick around until it was gone.

Even though there were times when it was tempting to let OCD blow away those relationships that weren't strong enough to hold, we didn't follow that path. Instead, we pulled Ray's OCD as far underground as we could where its effects would be less visible. We hid it as best as we could; we didn't talk openly about it; we did whatever we could to keep his symptoms from view; and we pretended it didn't exist around those who weren't willing to help us. Why we did this instead of just letting it rage in full view and taking our chances isn't easy to explain. I think it was because we learned early on that to let certain relationships go wouldn't be as easy as cutting a rope and watching them blow away. We saw that these relationships wouldn't go away but would remain in place, stubbornly refusing to budge. And unfortunately when this happened, it made it even harder for Ray and I to fight off his OCD. Some around us didn't just sit quietly by and watch us wrestle with the OCD but instead, raged back at us, yelled at us, made us doubt ourselves, and even tried forcing us down pathways we knew weren't right. They became yet another obstacle for us, so we decided that we had no choice but to find detours around them. If they weren't going to leave and weren't going to help us, then we needed to keep OCD as far away from them as possible.

Ray has some further insights into why some people around us couldn't help us as much as we would have liked.

ΔΔΔΔ

I can understand why some people who could have helped me more couldn't find ways to do it. Some of these people are only now beginning to understand my OCD years after my mom and I had successfully dealt with my sexual obsessions. Others, however, understood at the time that OCD was real and dangerous, but they also understood that it was something that required too much of a time commitment for them to really get involved. Furthermore, my OCD probably frustrated them as much as it did me, and this resulted in pushing them even further away from me.

Only a specific set of people can be relied upon to help someone fight their OCD. To fight OCD is a full time commitment because every compulsion and obsession has to be scrutinized and revoked. My mom had to be constantly on guard against my OCD, and this is why I made so much progress. To have the drive to help someone who is struggling with OCD, you half to have an enormous heart and uncommon generosity.

I do not blame those who did not help me with my OCD. To help me, my mom had to leave her job as a doctor in order to devote the time needed to deal with my OCD. This isn't something that everyone can do. What they can do, however, is to acknowledge the pain and suffering that OCD causes. For a long time, there were those around me who never really grasped the idea that I was dealing with OCD, and I do not think they had any clue as to how serious it could be. Because of this thinking, these people would often tell me that I needed to be stronger or would tell me that I could get over my problems if I just worked harder at it.

It would have helped me a lot during the time my OCD was bad if I had had some more acknowledgement of how tough OCD is and of how sometimes the weird actions you take are a product of OCD. I think this is one of the reasons why a lot of people do not get over their OCD. When people constantly think of you as bizarre and do not understand that you are dealing with OCD, it makes it difficult to interact with people. In fact, I avoided some people because I did not want them to think of me as weird. However, when I slowly began teaching those around me about my OCD, I became more comfortable and started spending more time with them.

ΔΔΔΔ

As Ray's OCD improved and his life returned to normal, the stresses on our personal relationships lessened. We have strove to reconnect with those who seemingly abandoned us and have tried to forgive them for their ignorance even though they have yet to acknowledge their mistakes and the pain they caused us. Ray has done this beautifully; he has gone on and has allowed certain personal relationships to reform and strengthen. He holds no grudges and wants to forget the past and all the negativity that resides there. I, however, have not been so successful in letting go but have tried to follow Ray's lead in this area. I still harbor anger and sometimes, have to fight to keep it in check. Many times, I have wanted to stand in the faces of those we most needed and who let us down and scream, "Where the hell were you when we needed you? Didn't you see what Ray was up against? We needed help, and you just turned away. How do you expect me to forgive and forget what you did?" But, I don't. It wouldn't help Ray rebuild his life after OCD if I keep digging up past regrets and keep stressing our worn relationships. The mature part of me knows that Ray is right and that we both need to move on, but the emotional part still needs convincing. Perhaps someday, I will grow up and let this go. I just can't do it yet.

If anyone had asked me to lay down money and bet on the personal relationship that I thought would most likely dissolve during Ray's OCD, I would have said, "That's easy. It's Ray's and mine. There is no way that Ray will want to talk to me again after all this or spend time with me." Throughout Ray's therapy, I was the one pushing him to do what he most feared, forcing him to keep going when he wanted to quit, keeping OCD up front in his life when he most wanted to avoid it, and refusing to help with his compulsions, those things that he knew for sure would give him comfort. Many times, I was the OCD-fighting bitch from hell, and Ray had to do what I commanded. Who wouldn't hate me when I was in that role? Sometimes, I couldn't even stand myself. And, I wondered if Ray would ever forgive me for the pain I caused him even though enduring that pain was what finally forced the OCD out of his life.

Turns out, I didn't need to worry. Ray not only has forgiven me but thinks that our relationship is stronger because of our OCD experiences. When I read what Ray had written regarding our relationship, I melted into a mushy pile. Truth was, I didn't know for sure what he would write about this subject. But, I was prepared to hear something painful and even share it, if that was what he thought.

ΔΔΔΔ

Because of our experiences with OCD, my mom and I have become very close. The reason for this is because of the nature of exposure and response prevention therapy (ERP). When doing ERP, I had to tell my mom my most embarrassing thoughts. Because of this experience, I can tell my mom anything that bothers me without fearing her judgment.

I know that my mom gave up a lot in order to help me get through OCD (her time, job, and independence) and for that I am forever grateful and thankful. I wish that I could somehow repay the enormous favor that my mom did for me, but I do not think there is anything that I could do to equal what she did for me.

The best thing I know to pay her back with is to never let OCD bother me again. In fact, this is one of several cognitive methods I use to battle my OCD when I feel it overwhelming me. I remember that my mom has given everything to help me, and if I ever let OCD take over my life again, it will be a grave insult to all the hard work that we did to get over my OCD the first time. I also know that my mom will be there for me whenever OCD tries to rise up again, and this is a big reason why I keep her close.

It is sad as I look at my friends and examine the relationships they have with their parents. Many of my friends do not enjoy the company of their parents and in some cases, they even loathe their parents. I think that one of the reasons for this disconnect is that the parents and their children have never connected on a deep emotional level. Maybe most of the interactions they had consisted of either authoritarian commands or passiveness, and great relationships cannot build on such interactions. My mom and I, however, ended up on a different path. We took on what I feared most and

275

together, embarked on a journey to defeat it. We struggled each day and sometimes almost gave up, but the companionship and the knowledge that we had each other was enough to keep going. I remember thinking that if I did not have my mom helping me through my OCD, then I doubt that I would have even tried to get over it.

As of now, I love spending time with my mom because she proved to me that she loves me by helping me fight OCD. I know that she cares about me and that provides enormous comfort to me throughout all walks of my life. I can look to her for advice, because I know she wants the best for me. And, I can even call her on the phone anytime of the day just to talk because I know that she truly loves me.

Not many parents have the opportunity to prove to their kids how much they love them and because of this, children often take their parents for granted. In a strange twist of fate, I am lucky in this regard.

ΔΔΔΔ

Shamefully, I have a confession to make: There were many times when I didn't want to be around Ray. Who would, right? OCD doesn't make us fun, companionable, or helpful. Instead, it forms us into a needy, whining, sniveling, and shaking mass. I was his mother, and he needed me, but yet, there were many times when I wanted nothing more than to get away from him. On some days, I couldn't stand to see the look on his face when an obsession was passing through his mind, the one where his eyes open wide, become unfocused, and where he frowns like he's just smelled something rotten. There were times when I also couldn't take listening to yet another confession or being asked to do something for him that a normal person would automatically do for themselves. I wish I had faced Ray's OCD with grace and patience. But, I didn't. There were times when I was awful to him, when I reacted strongly and negatively to the OCD, and when

I acted more like his enemy than his friend. Of course, I now regret these moments and am ashamed to even think about them, let alone admit them to others. My solace for these feelings was the realization that I'm not alone. Recently, a study was published which showed that parents often treat their OCD-afflicted kids with criticism and that they provide their non-OCD kids with more loving expressions. Of course, I still felt bad because of my behaviors, but at least, I knew that I wasn't the only one who had acted badly towards their child.

Even with all that was stacked against us, Ray and I still made it. We still talk often to each other, have fun when we're together, and most importantly (at least to me), he still turns to me when he's struggling. I hear about all his college woes, his uncertainties with friends, and his worries about his future. And, I am still involved in helping him manage his life. Recently, he made my heart soar when he said to me, "Thanks mom, I feel better now after talking to you. I knew you would say something that would help." In this instance, he had been beaten down by a barrage of difficult tests and was worried about his grades. After listening to Ray's worries, I looked for information that could be put together to help him reform a healthy perspective. I found syllabi for his courses, gathered up all the differing grading policies, punched some numbers, and then showed Ray how he could still get the grades he wanted. He had been too emotionally exhausted to see these paths but was grateful that I had found them.

I know that many, mainly those whose kids were lucky and didn't have to deal with a mental illness, would accuse me of being a "helicopter parent" and harangue me for being too involved with Ray. They would probably say things like, "He's a college student now. You need to let him be and find things out on his own. Stop babying him. You are doing him more harm than good by remaining so close to him." But, I have long stopped listening to those parents who were simply good enough, and whose kids thrived, not because they were so wonderful parents, but because they were lucky. Their kids didn't have OCD, or any other mental illness, that would force them to rethink their parenting strategies and to go down paths not traveled by most parents. And here's another observation: How well do most college students do on their own anyway? How many could use a little more parental involvement in deciding what classes to take, how to organize their time, or what activities to get involved in? Maybe if more parents stayed closer, asked a boatload of questions, and helped their kids form detailed plans, then there would be less drinking and drug use on college campuses, less depression among college students, and more students graduating on time. But, these are just my thoughts. What could I possibly know?

Whenever I start worrying about my level of involvement in Ray's life and wonder if it's time for us to cut our strong ties, I'm reminded about a metaphor that is often used to describe how different kids function in certain environments: Dandelions vs. orchids. Dandelion children, like the flower, bloom even in the most barren and harsh environments. Of course, they would probably do better and grow larger if given the opportunity to put down roots in fertilized and watered ones, but nevertheless, they can do OK wherever they land or whatever parents they were given. But, even with this amazing ability to survive, there's still one thing that they will always struggle to change: They're dandelions. Attractive, contributing, useful, but ordinary. Maybe with extraordinary effort, luck, and persistence they could bloom as something else, but chances are, they're destined to look like everyone else.

In contrast, there are the kids who are more like orchids. They wither without a constant source of enrichment; they require constant tending and care and are often amazingly difficult for their parents to understand how to help them. Their parents do all the usual things: Feed, water, love, talk, play, and educate, but yet their kid stubbornly refuses to bloom. It's only when their parents try something unusual or go against the usual parental dictums that they finally see a spark. Maybe they let up on the discipline or on their expectations for their kid's schoolwork. Perhaps they simply stop trying to push their kid and start listening to what their kid is saying. If they're lucky, it works, and their kid starts growing. Where once there was just barren soil there's now persistent growth and in time, there may even be something as beautiful and unique as an orchid. Not a dandelion, but something more exquisite and breathtaking.

I think that many who have mental disorders are like orchids. They don't have a chance to grow, let alone bloom, unless their environments contain specialized elements, and they receive constant and loving care. But, if they are lucky enough to land in the right environment that is tended by the right people, they do amazingly well and even better than most around them. I know that many would probably scoff at this idea and think I'm delusional. They might assume that I'm trying to comfort myself because my child has a mental disorder and that I don't want to assume the blame for him having so many problems. Or, maybe they think I'm being naieve, "Every mother thinks their kid is an orchid," they might say, "She's just stupid if she thinks her child is in any way special." Maybe they're right. I can be pretty stupid at times. I admit it. I can be as blind as any parent when it comes to my child. But in this case, I don't think so. Several experts have described the characteristics of these orchid children, and some scientists have even located a gene that may be involved. Unfortunately, this gene is also associated with mental problems, such as addictions and depression. In other words, in the wrong environment anyone who has this gene will probably suffer from a mental affliction whereas others who were lucky enough to have nurturing and creative parents will thrive and do even better than many of their peers.

Are all people who have OCD like orchids that will bloom

brightly once they find the right environment? It's hard to say for sure, but I think it's possible. I don't base this idea on wishful thinking or on a need to find something positive about my son having OCD, but on something I read in an OCD book, which had been written by an OCD expert. This expert suggested that OCD might result from an ineffective pruning of neuronal (brain) pathways that should normally be removed during certain times of development. (Several times during human development the brain undergoes massive reductions in all its connections.) But in addition to not removing the OCD pathways, other ones, which are involved in positive qualities, like intelligence and creativity, are also not pruned away. In other words, maybe those who have OCD maintain more brain pathways than normal, both the good and the bad. Needless to say, this idea is appealing. It means that even though those who have OCD may struggle hard and long to overcome their obsessions, they can accomplish incredible things once their OCD is under control. They can their use extra brain power to bloom like orchids, bright and brilliant.

So, what does all this have to do with Ray, his OCD, and our relationship? Simply this: I remain close to him even when others keep telling me to back off. I do more for him than what other parents do for their kids at this stage in their lives. I have not cut him loose, to swim or sink on his own and to learn those hard lessons of life that come with overt failure. This, I'm sure, will happen in time, but not now. At the moment, he does better with more care, not less. So, why shouldn't I stay involved? Dealing with his OCD has taught me to not let go, even when I see other parents cutting their kids loose. I learned how important it is to hold tight in spite of its social unacceptability because when I do, Ray pulls through his OCD or whatever mess his OCD has left him to deal with.

I don't know if Ray is more like an orchid or a dandelion, and I don't care. When we were struggling through Ray's worst days of OCD, I would have been happy just to have him show some growth instead of the constant withering that OCD was causing him. I would have celebrated a dandelion as greatly as the most magnificent flower ever to bloom. In fact, I would have celebrated any hint of green during that time. Any at all.

One final idea about the aftermath of OCD: After all that OCD has put us through, can I see any good to having had OCD in our lives? My answer to this is simple. No, not at all. I hate OCD with all my being and always will. I have personally experienced its destructions too many times to ever think that it has any redeeming qualities. I understand that others, who have suffered through mental illness, may think differently and feel that their struggles have made them better people. I just can't do it. I can't ever concede the idea that OCD has given us anything of value. To me, it's like asking me to praise my torturer because he made me stronger or was responsible for creating a goodness in me.

Ray, however, is more open to the idea that having dealt with OCD has given him some positive ideas about how to live a better life.

ΔΔΔΔ

OCD has affected me permanently in the way I look at life. Because of my OCD, I have learned that life is short and that too much time can be wasted worrying about frivolous consequences or possible shortcomings. I used to be hesitant in trying new things or in going to new places. I was this way because I feared that new and exciting experiences might stimulate my OCD and make it worse. Thus, I barely joined any clubs or other activities in high school and even as an OCD-free junior, I never attempted to make new friends. However, upon realizing the many opportunities that OCD has taken from me, I have become more eager to try out new things. I now love to travel, talk to any person I can find, and try out things I never would have had before. All in all, OCD made me realize that life is short and that full advantage of the good things must be taken if I am to have a good life.

OCD has not been a good thing in my life, but I have learned to make as much of an advantage of it as I can. I use the wisdom I have gained from battling OCD to guide my everyday life, from being more outgoing to giving people the benefit of the doubt for acting weird or being outlandish. But that said, OCD is something I wish had never come into my life, and I would never wish it upon someone else.

College

Give anyone with OCD enough time and support, and they can do anything. They can become doctors (I did), lawyers, scientists, journalists, teachers, business owners, political leaders, or great parents. Any vocation is within reach of those who have OCD. There was a time, however, when I couldn't imagine thinking this. When Ray was at his worst, there was little hope that he would ever achieve independence. I had accepted the idea that I might have to provide long-term support for him and had started formulating my future plans to accommodate him. I had even thought through several business scenarios where we would work together. Maybe we could operate an organic farm on our property or could start a publishing company where he could help me with the writing, editing, and distributing of books. My goal with all these ideas was to find a place for Ray where he would feel safe, useful, and in control.

Fortunately for Ray, his OCD responded quickly and thoroughly to his therapy. When we realized that Ray's future was now back in our hands, we started thinking about his next step: College. Even with all the havoc that Ray's OCD had caused him through high school, he still had a decent record (all A's and B's). But, we knew that many colleges and scholarships weren't available to him because of holes in his record. After perusing several college application forms, I immediately saw where he would have problems. There were many lines that needed filling out (ie, for extracurricular activities, community service, job experience, and names for references) but would have to be left blank because Ray had nothing to put down. He had been too busy dealing with his OCD.

I searched in the college applications for a space where we could describe Ray's OCD and to explain why he couldn't be in many extracurricular activities, hold a job, or volunteer in the community.

283

We needed to explain that Ray had used his after school hours, evenings, weekends, and even vacations to deal with and overcome his mental illness. We also wanted to explain that dealing with a mental illness like OCD is exhausting and that anyone who has OCD often has to spend their energy handling its many demands. But, I couldn't find anywhere on those college applications where Ray could put his experience with OCD and show how he had spent his time overcoming it.

An additional problem with Ray's college applications was that many of them required letters of recommendation. Because Ray had decided that he wanted his teachers to treat him like any other student and not one that needed special consideration, he had never disclosed his OCD to any of them. He wanted to feel that he had achieved his grades in the same fashion as other students and not because a teacher felt sorry for him. Maybe this approach wouldn't work out for every student who has OCD, but it was the right one for Ray and his teachers. The problem that this approach caused Ray, however, was that his teachers didn't understand many of his OCD behaviors and had attributed what they saw to a lazy, difficult, and immature student. As a result, they did what most teachers would do in these situations, they penalized Ray. When he failed to get to class on time because he had stopped to wash his hands, he got detentions. When his obsessions were swirling so fast in his mind that he couldn't pay attention, he was yelled at. When he didn't hear the teacher's instructions because his OCD was too loud in his head, he was publicly ridiculed for not knowing what to do. He also had been reprimanded for playing computer games in class, an activity he sometimes resorted to in an attempt to distract his mind from overwhelming obsessions. I can understand why his teachers resorted to these actions; they viewed his behaviors as a sign of immaturity that needed punishment and not for what they really were: A kid fighting, and often losing, his battle with OCD. But, because Ray insisted on his teachers not knowing about his OCD and because his OCD caused obvious problems in the classroom, these teachers were not ones who could provide Ray with useful letters of recommendation.

Our solution to the problems presented in many college applications was simple: Find an application that didn't require so much proof of success or teacher referrals. In the end, Ray decided to attend a local state university, which was in the same town as his high school. For a while, he wasn't thrilled with this idea, especially after watching some of his classmates gain entrance into the top universities in the country. At one point, he even convinced me that he should try applying to one of these universities, but of course, he was turned down. And honestly, I regretted that application the moment it was turned in. Even though his record had markedly improved during the last year of high school, he still had the gaping void of the first years. Also, I had become disillusioned with the whole process. I knew what Ray could do; I had seen him work hard to overcome his OCD. Maybe this wasn't proof enough of his abilities to those on college admission committees, but I no longer cared. Ray could achieve success anywhere he landed.

Even if Ray had been admitted to one of the coveted universities, I might not have let him go. OCD can turn wild again under times of stress and what is more stressful for an eighteen-year-old than moving away from home, dealing with new roommates, attending difficult classes, handling their finances, keeping their clothes clean, and feeding their bodies? And, they are expected to accomplish all this without their well-established support systems. Many college students stumble during their first semester, and for those who have OCD, it's even more difficult.

My concern was that if we weren't careful in Ray's college planning, OCD would find a way to take hold again. I worried that a college environment would prove fertile for OCD's regrowth in Ray. But, how to prevent this fear from coming true? Here's Ray's version of how we planned for his college experience.

ΔΔΔΔ

All high school students feel apprehensive when they think about college for the first time. And, when the time comes for your parents to move you to your college and help you unpack your overloaded suitcases and when you begin sifting through maps to find the locations of your classes, chances are you will pine for the predictability of life with your parents.

Some students fail, and some students thrive in college. What determines success or failure depends on many things, but I think that one determining factor is the management of stress (of which there are many underlying components). This isn't easy for most to accomplish, but now imagine that you are a teenager who has OCD and who has been thrown into this chaotic world where everything you once relied on for support may be hundreds or even thousands of miles away.

I have OCD and am now in my second year of college. Throughout my first year, I watched my fellow students both succeed and fail. Fortunately, I was among those who succeeded. I have concluded that the difference between those students who drop out of college or get bad grades and those who do well in college depends on how well a student can control what is going on around them and how well they can get things done. And, for those of us who have OCD, this control and organization is even more important to our success.

For those of us who have OCD, we face a whole gamut of potential setbacks that might ultimately force us to drop out of college and return to our distraught parents. Some of these setbacks include the exacerbation of current OCD-related symptoms, the development of new symptoms, or the relapse into old symptoms. Both my mom and I knew that my OCD could worsen during college and could even force me into quitting. With this in mind, we dedicated extensive thought on how best to help me control my stress and to keep my OCD as far back as possible during the semester. We acknowledged that the lower my stress was, that not only would my grades be better, but my OCD symptoms could be maximally mitigated.

My OCD had mostly been eradicated by time I graduated from high school. But, I know that if OCD had remained in control of my life that my mom would not have allowed me to attend college. I had gained this freedom by undergoing multiple sessions of therapy over about two years. In addition, I had even been successful in coming off all medication. Only at this point, were my mom and I comfortable with the idea of me going to college. However, the fact that OCD often flares during times of significant change or stress was something we had to consider. We knew that my OCD could rear up and cause me significant trouble if we didn't carefully plan. Therefore, my mom and I concentrated on putting me into college under the most stress-free conditions we could.

One of the most important decisions we had to make was what university to attend. For several years during high school I didn't think about college at all; my mind was too busy dealing with OCD. Unlike many of my fellow classmates who were actively working towards their futures, I was mired in obsessions. And, when I had finally beaten my OCD back and had retaken control of my life, I realized that I had fallen behind in many ways. Because of OCD, I had missed out on many important experiences in life and had failed to build the type of resume that certain, topflight universities require. I also wanted desperately to smack OCD back in the face by going to some far away, expensive, and prestigious school – almost like an ultimate retribution for the years OCD had taken away from me. I did not want to settle for what I considered a lesser school because I also had this desperate urge to prove

287

to everyone around me that I was capable of being among the best.

In time, I was convinced that academic excellence can happen anywhere and that it would be under my control to excel wherever I went. My mom also reminded me about OCD's sheer tenacity and that my OCD could resurface under times of great stress. If I was somewhere far away, then I might not receive help in time to keep my OCD from getting much worse. Therefore, I decided to attend a university that was close by and one that I had already previously taken classes at. In retrospect, my decision worked out well. The small exacerbations of OCD that I had were quickly stamped out; I kept my stress levels under control; and I finished the year with great grades. Also, after learning even more about how to deal with my OCD backlashes and after gaining confidence in my academic ability, I can now set my sites on the higher ranking schools if I decide to attend graduate school.

After deciding where I should go to college, we then focused on where I should live during college. Initially, I was leaning towards the idea of living in a dorm. I liked the possibility of developing close friendships due to the proximity of people within the dorms and the promise of a great social life. My parents suggested otherwise, believing that dorm life actually raises stress and instead of promising a good social life, may inhibit one. Following their advice, I decided to live off campus in a condominium that is a ten minute walk from my classes. We had also talked with older students who had lived in the dorms during their first years in college, and many of them said that if given a choice, they would have definitely chosen not to live in the dorms.

Living in the condominium, away from all of the fiascos and craziness of the dorms, was essential for me in handling my stress in college and subsequently, in handling my OCD. I could study efficiently without the distractions that dorm living entails and not have to migrate to a library to find peace and quiet. I also didn't have to worry about getting adequate sleep. Some of my friends, who had lived in the dorms, had party-all-night roommates who would often stumble into their rooms around 3:00 a.m. in the morning. Being chronically sleep deprived because of inconsiderate roommates was not something I was willing to risk. Of course, many students do just fine in the dorm environment, but I knew that I would be taking a chance that my OCD might reappear in force if I wasn't careful in managing my living environment.

I also attribute my staying OCD free to the close contact I maintained with my family. Even though college is often thought of as the time when we should gain our independence and leave the nest, I think it is important to keep our family and support systems close whether we have OCD or not. Several times throughout the first semester of college, I felt OCD slowly descend upon me. Although I could often, but not always, pinpoint my anxiety-inducing thoughts as OCD, I sometimes couldn't quickly overcome them. In these cases, I would either call my mom or would meet with her. I could do this because my university is close by my home. We would then talk through my thoughts and on occasion, we would need to develop a short therapeutic treatment. But for most times, simply identifying my worries as OCD was good enough.

One example of when OCD tried to get the better of me happened about halfway through my first college semester. I began having endless thoughts over a weekend that I had failed a calculus test despite the fact that I inherently knew that I had done well on the test. Even though I knew the answers, did not struggle through any part of the test, and even finished significantly early, I obsessed over the possibility that I had failed the test and that my life would be ruined. For me, that weekend was practically ruined by my obsessive thoughts. I even worried that future employers would see that single failed test and would not employ me. It was like my OCD had convinced me that by failing one test I would be forever viewed as incompetent and worthless. Despite being a veteran in dealing with OCD, I could not immediately recognize these thoughts as OCD. I ended up calling home to discuss my thoughts and ask for reassurance that I had done well on the test. Immediately, my mom saw that these thoughts were from OCD and then quickly constructed a therapy exercise for me. In this exercise, I repeatedly recited the idea that I would, in fact, fail not only this test but every other test in my college career and that my life would go to shambles in a very short time. Soon, I was anxiety free, and my obsessions were gone. I think that if I had proceeded to college without this kind of immediate backup to help me deal with my OCD flares, I could have relapsed back into serious symptoms.

In addition to times of stress, my OCD sometimes creeps back into my life during spans of downtime and relaxation periods such as spring and summer breaks. When my mind has a chance to wander freely and is not actively engaged in homework or classes, it sometimes strays towards OCD-like thoughts. One example of this occurred during the beginning of a summer break. Shortly before the semester had ended I had begun experiencing some minor problems with my sleep. During this time, I was routinely waking up every night at around 3:00 a.m. but was immediately able to fall back asleep. However, I began obsessing that because of these nocturnal awakenings, I would amount to nothing in my life because I would be chronically sleep deprived. I even compulsively talked about this to my mom who suggested that this thinking was the result of OCD and was not based on any reality. Once I accepted this as a possibility and started finding ways to keep my mind engaged in more useful activities, my obsessions went quickly away. What this minor episode reminded me of is that OCD might try to come back during periods of downtime and that I need to remain aware of this tendency. For those of us college students who have OCD, it might mean that we need to stay busy during these periods. We need to get a job, apply for internships, train for a marathon, anything that does not allow OCD to get a foothold. I sometimes imagine that OCD is like a *colony of deadly ants that, given a chance, will consume you. If you are standing still, then the attack will be slow but steady, but if you are moving, the ants (ie, OCD) will never have a chance to catch you.*

I plan to continue using the strategies I have developed and to keep looking for new ones. As I go through college, I know that I will have to face many different types of stresses and find new ways to deal with those challenges. But, I am not afraid any more that OCD will keep me from succeeding in college.

ΔΔΔΔ

Even if Ray's OCD hadn't been tame enough for him to attend college right after high school, we wouldn't have given up on the idea. The active presence of OCD in one's life doesn't mean that dreams have to be abandoned, just postponed a little. Maybe the path to college, or anywhere else, will be more indirect and winding for those who have OCD. We might have to find alternate routes to get where we want, like a detour around a construction site. For college, there are many different ways to get there and stay successful once there. If attending college full time is too hard, a student could always start with one or two classes and work from there or attend a junior college for awhile. Even failure at college is never a permanent failure. Any student who has failed can always come back, start over, and rebuild again.

Stigma and OCD

In the U.S., we have made amazing progress in so many social areas. Today, we can boast that race, religion, sexual orientation, and gender are all areas that have seen unimaginable growth. It wasn't that many years ago when women didn't have the right to vote, when Catholicism was an issue during presidential campaigns, when homosexuality was considered a mental illness, and when African Americans were forced into riding the back of buses. With all this enlightenment of the past few decades, it amazes me that mental illness still remains surrounded by so much stigma. Many of us who have a mental disorder still don't feel safe talking about it and go to extreme lengths to hide it. Ray and I certainly did.

When Ray's OCD first came to life, I was careful in keeping it hidden from the outside world. I did this more by instinct than by any specific reason that I could state. Was I wrong in doing this? Maybe I was reacting to some out-of-date ideas and had failed to see that the world was much more open and friendlier to those with mental illness than I thought. Sadly, I don't think so and for proof of the stigma that still surrounds mental illness, we don't have to look very hard. Almost every week, a newspaper or magazine article, TV segment, or major internet site reports on some aspect of mental illness that shows how it's still something to be ashamed of. During a recent presidential campaign, for example, one candidate remained coy about her history of migraines and wouldn't directly answer any questions about this aspect of her health. Even though a migraine is a neurological diagnosis and not a psychiatric one, it's often associated with psychiatric conditions like depression and anxiety. Plus, suffering from frequent migraines often suggests that someone takes medications for it, which is yet another dimension to stigma. If this candidate was uncomfortable revealing her history with a neurological condition, just imagine what lengths she would have gone to if she had something decisively more psychiatric, like OCD.

Every time a celebrity or politician backs away from public view and either refuses to state why or says something vague like, "I just want to spend more time with my family," my first thoughts are that they have some sort of mental illness and because of the stigma surrounding it are afraid to say so. Recently, for example, a congressmen suddenly disappeared from public view during a time when he was actively campaigning. His office refused to say where he was, which immediately fueled the rumor mill. Turns out, he has bipolar disorder and had been hospitalized for treatment. But, he obviously didn't feel comfortable revealing his diagnosis or where he was. In a stigma-free world, this wouldn't have happened, and his hospitalization for a mental illness wouldn't have been anymore newsworthy than if he had broken his leg or needed surgery. I would love if someday soon, a politician would stand up and tell the world, "Yes, I have OCD (or depression, general anxiety disorder, bipolar disease, or schizophrenia) and have been treated for it for many years. It doesn't affect my job performance more than a physical condition. I refuse to deny my diagnosis any longer and will answer any questions regarding it."

Because Ray kept his OCD hidden from most people, such as his teachers, coaches, and friends, he didn't experience any blatant discrimination. Even with this layer of protection, however, we still encountered stigma, just a more nuanced, softer version of it. After we had gotten through the worst of Ray's OCD, for example, we told some family members what we had been going through. They listened politely, shook their heads, said something sympathetic, but then looked visibly relieved when the subject of conversation changed. And after that initial conversation, we have never been asked how Ray's OCD is or how's he getting along with it. No one has ever asked for more information or in any way indicated to us that they understood what OCD is and how it had affected Ray. I doubt that this would have been the case if Ray had had a physical condition like cancer or had been in an accident. I can imagine the questions and concerns we would have encountered if we had been facing other problems. "How's Ray doing? Has he had any side effects to the medicines he's taking? How much pain does he have to deal with?" And, we might even have received support like, "It's really amazing how Ray is handling all this. He's really brave to facing these difficulties like he is. Tell him we're all thinking about him and rooting for him." Instead, we were met with silence and in that silence we heard shame, guilt, and embarrassment. We felt like we had become the family's dirty little secret that no one wanted to talk about. We had become our own version of, "Don't ask, don't tell."

Even the mental health community indirectly contributes to the stigma of mental illness. I understand why this happens; they need to protect their patients from the rest of the world and in most cases, they have no choice. We experienced this the first time Ray visited his psychiatrist. As we were filling out the necessary paperwork, it was clearly, methodically, and thoroughly explained to us that all records of his mental health visits would be kept separate from the rest of his medical records and that no one would readily have access to them. I think the receptionist spent more time on this issue than Ray's psychiatrist did on explaining the medication that he had prescribed during that visit. They obviously were doing this because mental health issues have yet to be accepted on the same level as other conditions. Otherwise, why wouldn't the charts be altogether in one place? We ran into a similar situation during one of Ray's follow-up visits with his psychiatrist. Ray had been scheduled to see the doctor in one of his satellite offices, which was closer to us. But when we got there, we had a hard time finding the actual office; we found everybody else: The gynecologists, the gastroenterologists, and the neurologists.

We finally stepped into the gastroenterologist's office for help, and they kindly directed us to the office across the hall marked "clinical services." Instead of clearly identifying themselves as psychiatry or even behavioral health, the mental health professionals were hiding behind a vague, confusing, and unhelpful sign. Apparently, the perceived stigma of mental disorders is so bad that we even don't want to be seen stepping into the office of a mental health professional.

Even after Ray and I started writing about OCD we still faced subtle hints about stigma and how it might affect us. Prior to the publication of each article, we were asked, "Do you want us to use your full names or should we use only your first names so that no one can identify you?" I know why this is asked, and I do appreciate it. And, I certainly don't blame anyone who chooses not to identify themselves on an article or blog they have written on their mental disorder. I even had a moment's hesitation prior to our books on OCD being published. Should we really throw caution to the wind and put our names on these books? Should we be more careful and not let the world know about our struggles with OCD? Would I someday regret being so open because it had negatively affected Ray? Maybe. But, I am also so tired of all the stigma surrounding mental illness and would only be contributing to it if I didn't face down my own fears, slap our names on our books, and see what happens. Wish us luck.

Each of us who has dealt with a mental illness knows that stigma still surrounds our condition and that it's better for us if we suffer quietly. Even though so much social progress has been made in other areas, mental illness continues to lag behind. Why this stigma continues isn't clear to me, but I imagine that the usual suspects are to blame: Fear, ignorance, and misinformation. Even those of us who suffer from a mental illness share a portion of the blame. We don't stick up for ourselves. In many cases, it's because we're too sick. When you are actively obsessing, compulsing, hallucinating, panicking, wrestling with mania, or are too depressed to even get out of bed, there isn't much energy left over to deal with an issue as large, complicated, and entrenched as stigma. We don't have the resources to pick up signs and march down the street for our cause. And when we do manage to regain our health, we often just want to join the masses and be normal. We want to have jobs, families, go on vacations, and enjoy life; we don't want to take on a social issue. We are also often behind in our lives and need to use all our resources to catch up. Ray once said to me when I first suggested to him that he become an advocate for those who have OCD, "I don't want to talk about what I've been through. I just want to put it all behind me and go on." I don't blame him. If I had any sense, I would have let him be and not insisted that we write this book.

The main way that those of us who have a mental illness contribute to the stigma surrounding it is by staying hidden. But who can blame us, right? There was time a time when we were grabbed, held down, zapped, or worse: Had an ice pick jabbed through our eye ball into our brain (the most efficient technique for performing a lobotomy). It was also not long ago when the cause of our ailments was thought to be possessions by witches or devils. More recently, we have heard that our sickness results from bad mothering or because we possess a weakness of will. We have also listened to others tell us that we aren't sick; we are lazy or malingers. If we would buck up, grow up, pull ourselves up by our bootstraps and just stop all our nonsense, then we would see that there's nothing wrong with us. With all this misinformation and idiocy swirling around us, we learn early on that it's best if we keep hidden. In fact, it's definitely safer and healthier for us.

Even though I appreciate how today's media has helped to explain, enlighten, and positively portray many aspects of mental illness, it still does one very damaging thing: It makes everyone scared of those who have mental illnesses. For most people, the first thing that pops into their heads when they think about mental illness is either the poor, dirty, and babbling homeless person they just passed on the street or the perpetrator of the latest shooting spree. And, how does anyone know about the latest murder, rape, shooting, or stabbing but via the media? The intensive coverage of these horrendous events often continues into the courtroom when someone inevitably invokes mental illness as the reason for why the crime occurred. Of course, these perpetrators are often mentally ill; maybe if they had received good mental health services when they were younger, they might not have done what they did. But, what isn't often said in these situations is how rare these events really are in the lives of those who have mental illness. It is a very small percentage of us who ever pick up guns and hurt others. Instead, most of us are cowering in our homes and trying desperately to fight off the enemy within. The only ones we ever hurt are ourselves.

In addition to the message that we are not dangerous I would also love to see the following idea displayed in big, block letters on a billboard in every city, town, and along all major highways: Mental illness is not funny. An obvious statement, right? But yet, our illnesses often serve as comedic fodder. In other words, we are laughed at, and it doesn't seem wrong to others that this happens. Comic strips, for example, commonly use mental illnesses as punchlines. For several months, I kept every comic strip from our local newspaper which used our illnesses for their laughs. OCD, hoarding (a form of obsession where an individual keeps unnecessary objects), agoraphobia (an extreme anxiety disorder when one fears outside places), Tourette's syndrome (a motor tic disorder commonly associated with OCD), and schizophrenia (a psychotic disorder where one has delusions and hallucinations) were all disorders that had been displayed as funny. Why does this happen so often? Imagine the outrage that would happen if cancer, epilepsy, diabetes, or stroke were used in a similar manner. Who would dare show someone having a seizure or parody the walk of a stroke victim just to get laughs? But when mental illness is used, there is no outcry. Instead of hearing the voices of our fellow citizens raised in our defense, we hear only smirks.

Maybe I could forgive the comedy writers who use mental illness for their material. After all, their job is to look at the world, find what is funny, and show it to the rest of us. Where my patience really runs thin, however, is with other professionals. Not long ago, I listened to a radio interview of an author who had just published a memoir on his experience with OCD. During the interview, the author was trying to explain some of his OCD symptoms and suddenly, there was laughter from the interviewer. The radio station was National Public Radio, and the interviewer was a well respected journalist who I had listened to many times and had liked. It broke my heart to hear that laughter. If this journalist didn't feel the need to restrain his outburst, then I doubt that many others would.

Yet another occasion where I witnessed OCD being laughed at was at a medical conference for professionals who take care of kids with developmental disorders. I was at a talk where a physician was discussing OCD. When she got to the point where she was describing the symptoms of OCD, she used an example that most of the audience found funny. It was like she was actually going for a laugh instead of discussing a serious clinical case. I wanted to jump on my chair, point my finger at her and scream, "How dare you laugh at us. You're supposed to be taking care of us and helping us get over our OCD. Our symptoms cause us unbearable pain and yet, you laugh at us." But, I didn't. I sat quietly, listened to the laughter, and wondered why it was happening. How could a physician so flagrantly find our symptoms humorous? I considered the possibility that I was just being too sensitive and needed to lighten up. Maybe laughter was one way in which these doctors handled the difficult cases they face every day. So, I listened carefully at all the other talks I attended; if humor is an accepted method of dealing with patients, I should hear it displayed throughout the entire conference. But, I didn't hear any further laughter. No one laughed when cases of autism, cerebral palsy, epilepsy, or mental retardation were discussed. No, the only laughter I heard was reserved for those who have OCD.

Those of us who have mental disorders are told in so many ways that our struggles aren't real. Our suffering isn't recognized or respected. And because of this, we often don't reach out for the help we need and the help that could save our lives. Even though Ray and I have found our way out of OCD, we worry that many others haven't and are afraid to ask for help because of stigma. They fear being ridiculed or shamed because they have repeatedly seen how those with mental illness are treated. Maybe Ray and I can't do much to change the attitudes of those who look down on us sufferers of mental illness. We would love to stand in their faces, grab them by their lapels, and shake some sense into them, but we can't. What we can do, however, is to try rallying those who are suffering. We hope that they can hear our voices, however faint, and know that they are not alone. There are millions of us out here. Many of us have even found our way to health and are now living productive lives in spite of the barriers and stigma we face. I know that many fear the stigma of having a mental illness, but I also think that this stigma is nothing more than a paper tiger that will one day be revealed for what it is.

∆∆∆∆

I think stigma still surrounds OCD because of a lack of understanding of what it really is. Sometimes, I wish that OCD was not so stereotyped as seen in shows such as "Hoarders" or the television series, "Monk." I also wish that OCD had a stronger impression with the general

299

public so that people can begin to understand how bad it really can be.

The lack of understanding of what OCD is can be annoying to those of us who have to deal with it. I also get annoyed when people without OCD attempt to empathize with my OCD by saying that they have OCD sometimes as well. I can remember one instance where I was meeting with my principal in high school to tell him why I had been late to so many classes. I explained to him that OCD was forcing me to wash my hands (I lied to him and told him I was afraid of germs and not sexual material for obvious reasons) and thus, I was showing up late to class. I explained to him how serious OCD is and how much it can ruin someone's life if not controlled. He responded by telling me that he has some OCD that makes him double check that the door is locked after he lies down in bed. My mom, who was meeting him with me, was furious on the inside. She did not let him know it, but my mom was dying to tell him that he does not have OCD and that his worries are frivolous compared to how bad mine were. Instances like these infuriate my mom and I because they demonstrate that people are not always able to acknowledge how bad OCD really is. And because of this fallacy, they may think that people with OCD are just weak willed.

I think that if the media covered OCD more accurately, the misconceptions surrounding OCD would not exist. If people without OCD were able to see OCD for how bad it really is, then the idea that people with mental disorders are weak willed would disappear. Instead, people with OCD (and other mental illnesses) would be seen as heroes for how much suffering they have to go through each day.

Others have sometimes described me through undesirable traits such as socially awkward, shy, weird, or stupid. But what people did not realize was that I was struggling with a monster that was very real to me but invisible to everyone else. When I finally got over my OCD, I felt like I had conquered the world. I looked at life in a new light of profoundness, but I also knew that *no one else understood that I had just destroyed something that almost killed me. How could I truly be a hero if no one (other than my mom, of course) saw me as a hero? This is what stigma does to those of us who have a mental illness. It makes us invisible; we have so few who are willing to share our struggles and also, our victories.*

I hope that someday, those of us who have a mental illness will face less stigma and receive greater empathy. I hope that we will be viewed as real people who are suffering and not with fear or with morbid fascination. If people could look at someone who is acting strangely and understand that maybe they have a mental illness, then those of us who suffer from a mental disorder will get the social support we need to get better.

Finding the Right Information on OCD

Throughout our time in dealing with OCD we have turned to many sources for help: Books (both those written by professionals and memoirs), mental health professionals, internet sites, people around us, television programs, and even fiction in the form of novels and TV/movie characters. And, we continue to look for new sources because we know that with something as complicated and dangerous as OCD one can never know enough. We suspect that someday, Ray's OCD will find yet a new way to surprise us, and it's best that we remain prepared. After looking under every one of these OCD-related rocks, however, we have learned one important thing: Be careful who you listen to and what you read.

I would have loved to say that everyone we turned to for help was kind, understanding, and knowledgeable, but that's not the case. In our personal lives, we ran almost immediately into the kind of ignorance that can cause widespread damage. In the beginning, I was often told things like, "It's all your fault Ray has OCD. If you just disciplined him more then he wouldn't have all these problems. You let him get away with too much with this OCD thing. He's manipulating you into doing what he wants. He's not sick; he's just using these behaviors to get out of doing his work." Lucky for us, I had enough medical training to know better. I knew from my years in pediatric practice that mental illnesses need real treatment, such as therapy and medications, and not simplified parenting skills, such as applying more discipline or teaching about responsibility. But even with this knowledge, I still felt the sting. Those words of blame found a way in and for a short time, I doubted myself. Maybe Ray's problems were my fault; maybe if I had spent more time with him, his OCD would never have happened; maybe I was such an awful parent that I had caused Ray such suffering. Of course, none of this is remotely true. I am as good as any parent.

Because of our experience, we decided early on not to reach out to those within our personal circle. They were too ignorant to help us and not willing to do much to correct their ignorance. We had no choice but to turn away, hide Ray's symptoms if necessary, and avoid as much contact as possible. At one point, we realized that we were willing to sacrifice all of our personal relationships. Our one goal was to save Ray, and anyone who got in our way of attaining that goal, regardless of their intentions, was cut loose from our lives. Even if Ray and I ended up with just each other and a handful of cats, we knew we would survive. We figured that once his OCD was taken care of, we could rebuild whatever relationships we needed, but until then, we needed all our energy and focus to fight off the OCD.

Also unfortunate for us was our choices of mental health professionals. They tried to help us; I have no doubt of that. They are not bad people. They just didn't know enough about OCD and its latest treatment (ie, exposure and response prevention therapy) to get Ray where he needed to go. And because of this, they got in our way and wasted our time. Instead of moving steadily towards mental health, we remained frustratingly mired in OCD land. We believed them when they said they knew how to lead us out. Why wouldn't we? They said they had the map and had told us that they had guided others who have OCD to the promised land of mental health. What I wished I had done instead of blindly trusting these professionals was to take control of Ray's treatment much earlier than what I did. I would have saved us precious time, effort, and money had I mapped out for ourselves where we needed to go and how we were to get there. It was only when I fully understood how OCD was effectively treated did I realize what we needed to do: Stop listening to those who didn't understand how to use exposure and response prevention therapy. I hope that many of our fellow sufferers of OCD have had better luck with their choice of mental health professionals than we did, but I suspect that many have fallen into the same traps.

Ray thinks that the loved ones of someone who has OCD are in the best position to provide help. Even though they may not know what to do in the beginning, they can learn, ask questions, and provide the necessary support.

ΔΔΔΔ

I am fortunate because I did not have to look far for help. My mom came to my aid when my OCD became serious. If I did not have my mom, I would never have had the drive to get over my OCD. The therapy to get over OCD was hard, and I would not have had the motivation to even try to get better by myself. For me, having my mom was imperative to my recovery. Without her, I might have eventually recovered, but it would have been slow, grueling, and exhausting.

In my opinion, the people who can really help someone with their OCD are their loved ones. For teenagers, I think that their parents are critical. I understand that many teenagers do not have parents capable of taking on OCD either because they are too busy or are unwilling to accept OCD as a real condition that needs treatment. Sadly, this is not ideal and is a situation that puts pressure on teenagers to handle their OCD alone, a situation scarier than I can imagine. My advice for any teenager who finds themselves in such a dilemma is to search for others who might provide help. There are professionals, such as psychologists or psychiatrists who specialize in OCD, that can help, and there are support groups that are available. And if these sources are not available, there are still many other ways to find help for OCD, such as reading books on OCD, looking at websites designed for those who have OCD, and joining online groups for OCD.

Most importantly, anyone who has OCD must never sit alone dealing with their thoughts. They have to let someone else know about

their obsessions or else a vortex of negativity and loneliness will en-
velop them. I do not think that I could have handled holding all those
thoughts within myself. If I had had no one to turn to or no one to talk to,
I may have given up. Even telling just one trusting friend, colleague, or
teacher can lift a huge load from someone who is struggling with OCD.

ΔΔΔΔ

Where I found a treasure trove of OCD information was via reading. I have long lost count of the number of books on OCD that I have read (some of them more than once). Of course, some books were more helpful to us than others, and I suspect that each of us who read these books get something different from them. After all, we are all at different places with our OCD; some are new to the diagnosis and need to start at the beginning; some have had OCD for years but are new to seeking treatment; and some might have successfully fought back their OCD but still need to fully understand what it all meant. Because of these different situations, I would hesitate to recommend any specific books (even this one) to my fellow sufferers of OCD. I simply don't know enough about anyone's specific needs to feel comfortable saying, "You simply must read ...... It will answer all your questions." But that said, I would like to give some general advice on OCD books. I hope it helps.

With regards to the books written by the professionals (ie, those who are specifically trained to deal with OCD), I suggest that those who have OCD read a couple of them. They generally give a good overview of what OCD is and how to treat it. In other words, these books are a good place to start. As to which ones to read, I don't have any specific recommendations; the ones I have read were similar in ideas and form and any would do fine. With regards to memoirs written by those who have OCD, however, my advice is different:

Read every one of them. I have read every one of these books I can find and continually troll for those I have somehow missed. Many of our fellow sufferers of OCD have bravely and openly penned their stories, and I hope that many more such books are forthcoming. Several of these memoirs have been published by large companies and have been expertly written and edited, whereas others have less polish. Regardless of form or appearance, each of these books has taught me something about OCD. Through the words of these authors, I have learned much more about OCD than I have from any other source.

In the last several years, fiction writers have also discovered OCD, and there are now several books that have main or side characters that deal with OCD. Sometimes OCD is upfront and driving in these stories and sometimes it's just along for the ride. Several of these books are helpful to those who have OCD (in my opinion) and show us characters who bravely face their OCD and who fight their way through the many obstacles that OCD places in their lives. But, many others don't. In several books, OCD was shown, not as the painful and soul rendering condition it really is, but as a quaint and cute personality quirk. In other books, the true horror of OCD is revealed and expertly described, but there is little hope for recovery in them. As hard as I tried, I couldn't find any solace in these books and was often depressed after reading them. There was even one fiction book that I would love to put a label on, "If you have OCD, please don't read this book because it might cause your OCD to worsen." In this book, a teenage character admits to having obsessions regarding harming others (a common type of obsession) and subsequently, finds herself talking to the police and eventually pursued by fanatics who are out to harm her. If I had read this book when Ray was first dealing with his sexual obsessions, I would have panicked and probably vowed never to talk openly about what we were facing.

With regards to OCD resources, I wish that I could give more solid advice. I would love to tell my fellow sufferers of OCD, "Read book A first, followed by book B, go to websites C and D, email or call persons E, F, and G, and if you still need more information, read books H-L. And at all costs avoid books, websites, and people, M-Z." But, I can't; no one can. We are all too diverse in our OCD for one educational plan to ever suffice. My best advice for all of us who deal with OCD is simple: Never stop learning about OCD. Because when you do, it might just find yet another way to catch you off guard and take over again.

Endings

Ray's Thoughts:

I think back on my life, and I cannot help but feel regret. I remember what a sad teenager I was, struggling through life when I should be having all the fun in the world. For a while, OCD took from me what was truly mine: My life. In return, it left me with almost nothing. But, OCD has also left me with a deepened sense of pride and ambition. Who else can claim that they have gone through something as tough and horrible as OCD, and more incredibly, come out of it thriving? I have learned many lessons from dealing with OCD, and for those I would not trade for all the money, social status, and fame in the world.

Sadly, OCD is the ultimate destroyer of the sense of self. The guilt that OCD causes stems from doubting many of our thoughts, and we have to repeatedly convince ourselves that we are not bad people, that we will not get sick, or that we did not kill someone with our car on the way home. During the worst of my OCD, I questioned every little, nuanced gesture I made, any small talk I engaged in, and even the very steps I took down a hallway. I worried that some small body movement I had made wasn't innocent but was one that had alerted a girl near me that I had intentions to molest her or that by shaking someone's hand I was engaging in some kind of sexual pleasure. I could never convince myself that any action I took was morally right. I feared myself more than anything.

Even today, I sometimes wonder if an action I took was the right thing to do and may spend time worrying about it. But, does this mean that I am forever doomed to live afraid of my own shadow? Will I ever become a truly confident person and attain my true happiness? I am confident that the answer to these questions lies in a philosophy of acceptance that I have recently adopted. I have now come to the conclusion that OCD amounts to nothing more than a fly on the wall. It took me many hours of contemplation to reach this conclusion, but it has helped me through the times when I can feel the doubt closing in on me. This lesson is invaluable to me because it can also be applied to other, non-OCD situations that I face in life. I also now view life as a journey filled with mistakes and uncertainties that will all be worked out in time.

I know that anyone who can control their OCD will be ready for any task they face in life. OCD does nothing but cause doubt, sometimes without relent. But if OCD can be controlled, then nothing is ever to be feared again because one's worst fears have already been conquered. I have accepted my OCD as a challenge, knowing that if I continue to meet this challenge then I will become a better and stronger person.

My final thoughts to my fellow sufferers of OCD are these: If OCD has you down, the way out of it is to treat it as a challenge. Just know that if you can beat OCD, you are ready for anything. If you can beat it, you have defeated your ultimate fear and are now free to take on any challenge that ever comes your way.

ΔΔΔΔ

My Thoughts:

It was tempting to end this book by saying something inane like, "We hope our words have made a difference. We hope that we have helped others who have OCD along their way. We want those who have OCD to know that they are not alone and that there are many others with OCD and who can help." All these words are true, of course. We really do hope that we have helped in some way. But, I also wanted to end this book with something more substantial, something that I wish had been given us when we needed it the most: A voice. When we were struggling with Ray's OCD, we couldn't find our voice to tell others what we needed to. Sometimes, we wanted to ask for help but were afraid to and some-

309

times, we simply needed to tell someone to "shut the hell up" because they were causing us more trouble than helping us. Here is my attempt to provide, at least partially, a voice to our fellow sufferers of OCD. Initially, I wasn't sure how to do this but then decided that maybe the best way was to simply write some letters that were addressed to different groups of people and see if that worked.

Here I address several groups: The unbeliever in OCD (ie, those who simply refuse to understand that OCD is a real condition that requires attention and treatment), those whom people with OCD come into contact, maybe even on a daily basis (ie, teachers, coaches, mentors, friends, colleagues, and non-immediate family members), and of course, our loved ones, those saints who stick with us in spite of all we put them through.

Dear Unbeliever in OCD,

First of all, stop talking. Right now, just do it. You have no clue as to the damage your words and actions have already caused and are currently causing. Do you even realize that some of that damage may already be irreparable? You may feel insulted by my forwardness in taking this approach with you, but I don't care. It's important that you understand how dangerous your ignorance is.

I don't have the time and patience to understand why you don't think that OCD is a real disorder like a physical illness is, why you dismiss the suffering of those who deal with it, why you think that those who have it have done something to deserve it, or why you think that someone with OCD can just get over it if they really wanted to. Maybe I should have more sympathy towards you and try to show you your errors. But admittedly, I don't think I can. I resent you too much. In fact, I despise you for the harm you have caused to those who suffer from OCD.

By your actions and words, you have done much damage.

There are those around you who are truly suffering and who need help. Their pain is intense; their lives are in turmoil; and they are in danger. But yet, you treat them like they are silly children who just need more discipline or a weakling who just needs more backbone. Maybe you think they are acting the way they do because they are trying to take advantage of you or to not take responsibility for their lives. This is wrong. No one who has OCD wants it, and everyone with this disorder is in pain.

The suffering OCD causes is real. You have yet to accept this and rarely hesitate to let your thoughts known. But your words have impact; there are those around you who are listening to you and who are taking your words to heart. Instead of looking for treatment for their OCD, they are berating themselves for their weakness in failing to deal with their condition. Instead of understanding that what they have is a legitimate disorder that can be treated, they are quietly suffering through each day. Instead of reaching out to the OCD community (via support groups, internet sites, or attending conferences), they are struggling by themselves to understand what is happening to them. Even if you don't think you can ever accept OCD as a real disorder, you can at least, stop spreading your ignorance and give those around you a chance for hope.

Someday, you will know what it is to suffer. Everyone does; this is part of the human condition. Your body will give out; a loved one will suffer or die before they're ready; or a child of yours will face an uncertain future. Suffering comes in an endless number of ways, and when it happens to you, you will need help and support. If you're lucky, you won't have to face your fears alone but instead, you will have an array of people around you who are willing to fight for you and who believe enough in you to find what you need. One of these people might even have OCD and is someone you now shun.

I doubt if my words will reach you and convince you of your ignorance. But in the chance that this letter has made a difference in your thinking, I will provide you with ideas on what you can now do. First of all, apologize to those you may have hurt and if necessary, drop to your knees and beg for forgiveness. Tell those who you have hurt that you were wrong but are now ready to start making amends. Second, start learning about OCD as fast as you can. You have a long way to go with regards to understanding what OCD is so the sooner you start the better. There are many books, websites, and videos that can help you in this regard. Third, do whatever that is in your power to lessen the pain of those who have OCD. It could be something as simple as cooking a dinner, babysitting, running some errands, taking on extra household chores, or simply sitting down and talking. Knowing that someone is around who cares enough to help can make all the difference to someone who is struggling.

Think you could do, at least, that much?

This is all I have to say to you.

Sincerely,

Joni St. John

Dear friends, teachers, coaches, mentors, non-immediate family, and anyone else in our lives who we didn't tell about Ray's OCD,

Hello. There is much I wish to tell you and explain to you regarding my son's condition, obsessive compulsive disorder (OCD). I suspect that you have seen parts of his OCD and most likely, didn't know what it was or what to do about it. I'm sure that there were times when you noticed his red, chapped hands and wondered why his parents weren't fixing it. Or, why he often seemed distracted and unable to focus or do what was required of him. Maybe you have even thought that he was rude or arrogant because he wouldn't respond to your questions or make eye contact with you. All of these behaviors, and many more, resulted because of his OCD and not because he was arrogant, willful, or disdainful of those around him.

First of all, let me explain that OCD, while a mental illness, is not dangerous. You and those around you are not in any danger from someone who suffers from OCD. It is not those who have OCD in our community who take up guns and kill others. They do not steal or rape. The only ones that are affected from OCD are those who have it (and maybe their loved ones) and in most cases, they suffer quietly. In fact, many who have OCD try hard to make sure that no one around them knows about their condition.

As to what OCD is, it's simple to state but hard to describe. OCD is when someone has recurrent, unwanted and intrusive thoughts (obsessions), and to deal with the anxiety that those obsessions cause, they often perform compulsions. The example of OCD that is often used in the media is someone who obsesses over their fear of germs and tries to relieve their anxiety by constantly washing their hands. Unfortunately, the compulsions never relieve the anxiety that someone with OCD feels, and they continue living in fear until they receive appropriate treatment for their OCD.

Because my son lived in constant fear, he had many problems which at times, extended into your world. For this, I am sorry. Your lives are also filled with many obligations and problems, and I'm sure that you were often dismayed at the additional burdens my son's OCD caused. Maybe you found my son's constant requests and excuses difficult to understand or his awkwardness in your presence tiresome. Perhaps you asked him a question, fully expecting to hear a reasonable answer but instead, heard what seemed like pure nonsense to you. This is what OCD can do to someone, makes them nonsensical to others.

For many reasons, I didn't feel comfortable telling you about my son's OCD. I didn't know how you would react to him if you knew about his "thoughts." Maybe you would have understood and could have helped him through his difficult times. But, we weren't willing to take that chance. Even though you seemed like someone who cares about those around you, we weren't sure how you would react to something as difficult and unusual as OCD. There is still much stigma and misunderstanding surrounding mental illness and because of this, we remain careful as to whom we talk to about OCD.

As you read this, you might be wondering what you could have done to help my son or others who have OCD. First of all, don't be afraid to ask questions. Openly show your compassion and show others that you are willing to understand even that which is confusing to you. Many times, I wished you had taken my son aside, asked him if something was wrong and if there was anything you could do. Maybe he wouldn't have responded to you but at least, he would have known that you cared. You could also have spoken to me and asked me what was happening and together, we might have found ways to make my son's life a little easier.

But as it was, you said nothing. And on many occasions, your actions towards my son made his way even more difficult. He heard the frustrations in your voice; he saw the disdainful looks you often gave him; and he noticed the praise and respect you gave others but withheld from him. He so wanted contact with you and often craved your positive attention, but he didn't trust you enough to tell you what he was experiencing.

Secondly, learn about mental illness. There are many resources which explain what mental illness is and what it isn't. You may already think that your knowledge is adequate, but I know from talking with you that your knowledge is too superficial. Too many people think they understand what mental illness is because of what they have seen on television, videos, or have read in magazines. It may be too late for you to help my son, but I'm sure that there are other kids (and adults) around you who have a mental illness and who could use your help and understanding. Please strive to understand them, reach out for them, and help guide them through their struggles.

Third, be an advocate for those who struggle with mental illness. I am not asking you to give up your time, money, or much of anything. Only this: If you hear others talking negatively or laughing at those who have a mental illness, please say something. Tell them that they are wrong to say such things and how they are hurting those who are already in tremendous pain. Tell others around you that mental illnesses are real, life threatening, and that people who have them need compassion and help.

I hope that what I have said in this letter touches you and that you have not taken any offense to my words. If you wish to continue this conversation, I would be happy to meet with you and talk more.

You know where I am and how to find me.

Best regards,

Joni

Dear Loved One (from one who suffers from OCD to their loved one),

How can I ever thank you enough for standing by me during my difficult times? I know how difficult I have made your life and how unfair it is for you to have this burden. I know that on many occasions you have looked at other families, who weren't affected by OCD, and felt jealous. You wanted their happiness, their ease in life, and their un-encumbered futures. But instead, you got OCD and the burdens it entails.

I wish I could tell you that OCD will someday be gone from your life forever, but that isn't true. Even if OCD fades for awhile, and it looks like it might never return, it often finds a way to come back. Sometimes it roars back to life and threatens to derail lives but more often, it sneaks in like a thief and steals something important before anyone realizes it has returned. But, I think that with your continued support and vigilance, OCD will have a difficult time finding its way back into our lives. And even if it does return, I know that with your help, we can force it back out again.

I know that many times you have wanted to quit and search for a less difficult life. There were many things you wanted to do or places you wanted to go but couldn't because OCD got in our way. There have also been many family gatherings and holidays that have been ruined because OCD wouldn't leave us in peace. For all this, I am truly sorry. You deserve so much more. I understand this and will try even harder to push OCD out of our lives so that we can have more enjoyment and peace.

I don't say this enough, but I'm thankful for your love and support. I see all that you do, every day even though there are times when it seems like OCD has crowded out all other thoughts. I see when you take on my work so that I can focus on dealing with my problems. I know that you have given up your free time to do extra parenting, running errands that I should have done, or simply holding my hand while I cried. You have also stood dutifully by me and protected my dignity during those times when my OCD was threatening to reveal itself. You know how hard this condition is to understand and that many others around us would probably turn away if they knew the strange and twisted thoughts that persist in my head. So many times, you have made the necessary excuses, created the sensical stories, and found an escape for me when I needed it. You have given up so much for me and for that, I will always be in your debt.

If it were safe to do, I would tell the world about your sacrifices, your loyalty, and your strength. I would put you on a podium and demand that you be nominated for sainthood or at least, given a Nobel-like prize. But in the world we live, it's not possible. There is still too much stigma and fear surrounding those of us who have a mental illness. All I can give you at this time is my gratitude, love, and undying respect. But, I will also promise you this: I will try with all that is in my power to not let your efforts be wasted. I will do whatever is necessary to keep OCD out of our lives.

You deserve this much.

Love,

Me

And finally, these letters:

Dear fellow sufferer of OCD,

Hello. Wherever you are in this world know this: You are not alone. I know that OCD often isolates us from others and convinces us that there are no others who are as messed up, ugly, bad, evil, smelly, or worthless as us. But that's not true; there many of us who have OCD and who have found ways to deal with it. So, wherever you are or whatever state your OCD is in, you can find help. Just be sure to ask. We, your fellow sufferers of OCD, are here, standing by with open arms. All you have to do is reach for us, and we will pull you in.

I'm sure you rarely hear this, but I think that you are among the bravest souls that I have ever seen. You face every day, even though you are scared; you get up not knowing what tricks your OCD will try; and chances are, you are picking your way through all this by yourself. What could possibly be a better example of courage? By living your OCD-laden life, you have proven that you are strong, probably stronger than most people around you.

I know that OCD has taken a lot from you, and maybe you feel that you no longer have much to give the world. This is not true. In fact, I think the world could use more people like you. You know what it is to suffer and how dark life can become with OCD in control. You can use that knowledge to help others who are struggling. Once you start taking back your life from OCD, you will see that your help is greatly needed. There are many others who could benefit from your experiences with OCD and who desperately need the hope you can give them.

I wish I could tell you that once you reach out for help that your ordeal is over, but that's not true. Dealing with OCD isn't easy, but you already know that. There's no magic pill we can take that solves our problems or surgery that we can undergo that corrects our faulty brains. But, there is a treatment (exposure and response prevention therapy (ERP)) that helps. That is the good news. The bad news, however, is that undergoing this treatment is not easy. It takes a lot of effort and stamina to really make ERP work. But, I know that you can do it; after all, you have shown your strength by living with OCD all this time, so why not use that strength to push OCD out of your life?

If there is one idea that I hope to convince you of it is this: ERP works. This therapy can give you your life back. But, you have to work for it. It's long and hard, and maybe there will be times that you are tempted to give it up and go back to your OCD-dictated life. Please don't. If you stay the course and keep pushing through, you will not regret it. In fact, you will be amazed as to how well ERP can push OCD out of your life. But this said, I need also to tell you that doing effective ERP can be tricky. It takes a right combination of effort, creativity, skill, and sheer persistence before its real effects can be felt. The important thing with ERP is to not give up on it. I'm convinced that it can help all who have OCD improve their symptoms and for some, it can come close to being a cure. It's that powerful.

For many of us who have OCD, getting started on ERP is hard. I can't tell you how to get started, that has to come from within, but what I can say is that you need to make the jump. Even if the ERP cliff looks ominous to you and even if you feel like you are about to fall, don't stop. Please take that first leap of faith. Trust those of us who have done it and who have taken our lives back. You need to jump. Really, it works. Many of us have done it and have no regrets at all. Just jump.

Now.

Please.

Trust me.

Warmly and with respect,

Joni

Dear Ray,

I have no idea how to start this letter. So many thoughts are swirling around my head that I am having a difficult time catching one and holding it long enough so I can write it down.

I had thought about starting this letter with the obvious, "I love you and will always love you no matter what happens in your life." But in our case, saying these words isn't necessary. You have long known by my actions what I feel for you. You have watched me go to the ends of the earth for you, stand by you when you had lost hope, and be there to reach for you when you needed my help. You know that I will always be here for you.

One thing I do need to ask of you: Please forgive me. There were times during your OCD struggles when I failed you. I lost my patience, yelled, and walked away when I shouldn't have. In the beginning, I failed to understand what you were dealing with and in my ignorance made it more difficult for you. I'm sorry for this. I regret it more than you can ever know. You had looked to me to help you but instead, I made your way even more difficult.

I'm very sorry that you have to deal with something as difficult as OCD. You did nothing to deserve this burden; you are just as good, competent, loving, and whole as anyone. It isn't fair that you had to suffer with OCD and that you had to struggle through each day while others lived so freely. I know how you have longed to laugh and experience life to its fullest. I have seen the pain in your eyes and have wanted nothing more than to ease that pain.

I know you probably won't believe this or think that my opinion here is only a mother's pride and not based on fact, but here goes: You are undoubtedly the bravest person I have ever known. To get through each day with OCD takes a strength few of us have or even imagine having. You have bravely faced each waking moment when your OCD was at its worst and have found ways to keep going. I admire you for this; I know how hard it was for you to take each step, but you did it. I have also witnessed your bravery during the intense times of your therapy. To be asked, repeatedly, and for days on end, to face that which you fear the most is not something for the faint hearted or weak. You accomplished this feat several times and for that, you have my admiration and respect.

I don't know what the future will bring us. I'm sure that we will have heartbreaks, will suffer, and will find times when our resolve weakens. I am also sure that OCD will try to take over our lives from time to time. That's how it works; we can never be completely rid of it. But, we can be certain of one thing: OCD can always be beaten back. We have proven this many times, and I have no reason to think that we won't continue in our success against OCD. As long as we stick together, keep calm, and believe in our abilities, success will be ours.

Many times, you have asked me if I was sorry that you had come into my life because of all the problems your OCD caused. I don't know if you have ever believed me when I have unwavering told you that "No, I would never give you up." There is no one on this planet who could take your place in my life. Had I wished, many times, that OCD had left you alone? Of course, but that has never meant I wanted you to be someone else. You are not defined by OCD; it's not who you are but only an obstacle that has gotten in your way and one that we have had to overcome.

I will end this letter now before you become impatient with me. You have often told me that I talk too much, especially when it comes to you. So, I will end with simply this.

I believe in you.

You are stronger than anyone I have ever seen.

If you ever need me, just look over your shoulder.

Love,
Mom

Notes

Part I - Our OCD Stories

Grandma's OCD Story

One suggestion that is often found in OCD books: The idea of staying busy to help deal with OCD symptoms can be found in many sources. One source, however, that addresses this concept well is: J.M. Swartz, *Brain Lock: Free Yourself from Obsessive-Compulsive Behavior,* (New York: Harper Perennial, 1996).

Ray's Compulsions

Ray started washing his hands: D.M. Clark, *Cognitive-Behavioral Therapy for OCD,* (New York: The Guilford Press, 2004).

Part II – Understanding OCD

Describing OCD

When asked about OCD: There are many definitions of OCD that can be found with a quick internet search. However, the underlying ideas are the same for each of them. The one used here is from: The Free Dictionary by Farflex (definition of obsessive-compulsive disorder). Available at http://medical-dictionary.thefreedictionary.com/OCD.

Introduction to Understanding OCD

When people who have OCD are placed in brain scanners: One source that shows an interesting scan that demonstrates how the brains of those who have OCD differ: J.M. Schwartz, *Brain Lock: Free Yourself from Obsessive-Compulsive Behavior,* (New York: Harper Perennial, 1996).

OCD and Genetics

Some have suggested that the cause of OCD is: A good review on the genetics of OCD is: E. Hollander, et al. (editors), *Obsessive-Compulsive Spectrum Disorders: Refining the Research Agenda for DSM-V,* (Arlington, VA: American Psychiatric Association, 2011).

If these same genes are active in our fellow creatures: A good review on the observation of OCD-like behaviors in other animals is: E. Hollander, et al. (editors), *Obsessive-Compulsive Spectrum Disorders: Refining the Research Agenda for DSM-V*, (Arlington, VA: American Psychiatric Association, 2011).

OCD and Environment

The ancient Greeks: A good review on the documented history of OCD is: I. Osborn, *Tormenting Thoughts and Rituals: The Hidden Epidemic of Obsessive-Compulsive Disorder*, (New York: Dell, 1999).

Are really saviors and kings: The idea that OCD might be tied into ancient behaviors is discussed in: J. Rapoport, *The Boy Who Couldn't Stop Washing*, (New York: Penguin Books, 1989).

OCD has been found in every culture: A good review on the observation of OCD in different cultures is: E. Hollander, et al. (editors), *Obsessive-Compulsive Spectrum Disorders: Refining the Research Agenda for DSM-V*, (Arlington, VA: American Psychiatric Association, 2011).

Reminded of a story: B. Carey, *A High-Profile Executive Job as Defense Against Mental Ills*, The New York Times, October 22, 2011; Health Section.

OCD and Comorbid conditions

The list of possible comorbid: Good reviews of the comorbid conditions that occur with OCD are: D.M. Clark, *Cognitive-Behavioral Therapy for OCD*, (New York: The Guilford Press, 2004) and E. Hollander, et al. (editors), *Obsessive-Compulsive Spectrum Disorders: Refining the Research Agenda for DSM-V*, (Arlington, VA: American Psychiatric Association, 2011).

Up to 2/3 of those who have OCD: E. Hollander, et al. (editors), *Obsessive-Compulsive Spectrum Disorders: Refining the Research Agenda for DSM-V*, (Arlington, VA: American Psychiatric Association, 2011).

Sexual Obsessions

OCD affects 1%-2% of the population: D.M. Clark, *Cognitive-Behavioral Therapy for OCD,* (New York: The Guilford Press, 2004).

We did find one book: L. Baer, *The Imp of the Mind,* (New York: A Plume Book, 2001).

Looked at sexual obsessions and OCD: J. Grant, et al, "Sexual obsessions and clinical correlates in adults with obsessive-compulsive disorder," *Comprehensive Psychiatry* 47 (2006): 325-329.

Part III – Treatment With Exposure and Response Prevention Therapy (ERP)

Motivation to do ERP

We use our reward pathway: P. Bloom, *How Pleasure Works: The New Science of Why We Like What We Like,* (New York: W.W. Norton & Company, 2010).

Finding Help For ERP

How many in the mental health profession fail: H. Brown, *Looking for Evidence That Therapy Works*, New York Times, March 25, 2013, Health Section.

When I made the decision to direct Ray's therapy: L. Baer, *The Imp of the Mind,* (New York: A Plume Book, 2001).

Additional ERP Sessions

About a priest, Father Jack: L. Baer, *The Imp of the Mind,* (New York: A Plume Book, 2001).

Final ERP Sessions

During the third session we ended up using three tapes. The actual tapes that were used in this   therapy session are as follows:

Recording # 1: I was walking through Walmart when I saw a pretty girl who appeared to be about 16. She was wearing very short shorts and wore a revealing shirt. I could see part of her breasts. I had an erection. I could feel something wet in my pants. In the bathroom, I saw wet semen in my pants.

Recording #2: I was walking through Walmart, and I saw a girl. She was wearing a shirt revealing her breasts. I could see she was wearing a black, lacy bra. She was also wearing short shorts and had a very sexy butt. I think she was the sexist woman I had ever seen. I got an erection when I looked at her. Later, when I was taking a shower, I thought about the sexy lady, I got another erection, and I masturbated. The semen washed away down the drain, and I felt happy.

Recording #3: I was at a party with some friends, and they were watching a pornographic movie. I stopped to watch for a long time. I watched a man and a woman having sex, and they were really going at it. The woman was on top of the man, and she was moving up and down. Her breasts were very big, and they were bouncing all around. They were both groaning and making a lot of noise. After a few minutes of this, they both had orgasms. Then, the movie showed another man and woman having sex. This time the man was behind the woman and was moving back and forth. The man ejaculated, and then fell over the woman's back. Then, the movie showed another couple. This time the woman was giving the man oral sex. Her mouth was moving up and down the man's penis, and he was groaning. When he ejaculated, his sperm got all over the woman's mouth. When I was watching this movie, I got an erection, and all my friends also got erections. I know this because we were all joking about it when we were going home. When I got home, I went into the downstairs bathroom to take a shower. I was thinking about the movie and all the naked women that I had seen. I got a big erection and masturbated while thinking about those women. My ejaculation was so intense that I got some of it on the shower wall.

We had also considered using an additional tape but didn't need to: I am walking down the street and I see a little girl. She walks away from her mother and goes down an alleyway where there is no one else. I follow her and quickly catch up to her. She turns and smiles at me but then looks afraid. I touch her body, and she cries at me to stop, but I don't. I can feel that I have an erection, and it feels intense. I reach under her clothes and touch her in a sexual way. When I get home I masturbate while thinking about the little girl, and it feels good.

Part IV – Additional Ideas for Treating OCD

Hank: An Unusual Therapy Aid

Now proven that over 50%: L. Schenkman, *Daydreaming is a Downer*, Science Now, November 11, 2010.

For children is critical: A good review of why children play is found in: J. Gottschall, *The Storytelling Animal: How Stories Makes us Human*, (Boston: Houghton Mifflin Harcourt, 2012).

Several magical characters: E. Kelly, *"Not Right" OCD and Interactive Storytelling*, OCD Newsletter, Summer, 2009.

Medications: Our Experience

One's brain slowly up-regulating: There are many books and articles that describe how medications work in the brain. I have included the reference where I first read about this information: P. Kramer, *Against Depression*, (New York: Penguin Books, 2006).

One popular book: P. Kramer, *Listening to Prozac*, (New York: Penguin Books, 1997).

Exercise

There are many studies at present that show how exercise affects the human brain. The ones listed here are only a random sample of the information that now exists in this area.

Exercise results in the birth of new neurons: G. Reynolds, *How Exercise Could Lead to a Better Brain*, New York Times, April, 18, 2012, Health Section.

College students also have improved memories: G. Reynolds, *How Exercise Benefits the Brain,* New York Times, November 30, 2011, Health Section.

Other Ideas

Researchers in neurobiology have looked: There are many sources which describe how meditation works in the brain. One good source is: R. Davidson, *The Emotional Life of Your Brain*, (New York: Plume, 2012).

Part V – Additional Issues on OCD

Aftermath of OCD

Showed that parents often treat: R. Nauert, *Traps Parents Fall Into When Caring For OCD Child,* Psych Central News, April 12, 2012.

Some scientists have even located a gene: W. Herbert, *On the Trail of the Orchid Child,* Scientific American, November 22, 2011.

Expert suggested that OCD might result: I. Osborn, *Tormenting Thoughts and Rituals: The Hidden Epidemic of Obsessive-Compulsive Disorder, (*New York: Dell, 1999).

Books

Many books (both nonfiction and fiction) have helped us understand OCD and how to deal with it. The following is a partial list of the books that have helped us deal with our OCD.

To our fellow sufferers of OCD: If you have written a book on your experiences but don't see it listed here, please forgive us. Please let us know, and we will find your book and promptly read it. We know that you have something to teach us.

B., J. (2008). *The Boy Who Finally Stopped Washing.* Cooper Union Press.

Baer, L. (2002). *Imp of the Mind.* New York: Plume.

Bailey, J. (2007). *Man, Interrupted: Welcome to the Bizarre World of OCD, Where Once is More is Never Enough.* London: Mainstream Publishing.

Bell, J. (2007). *Rewind, Replay, Repeat.* Center City, MN: Hazelden.

Bell, J. (2009). *When in Doubt, Make Belief: An OCD-Inspired Approach to Living with Uncertainty.* Novato, CA: New World Library.

Binstock, M. (2011). *Nourishment: Feeding My Starving Soul When My Mind and Body Betrayed Me.* Deerfield Beach, FL: Health Communications, Inc.

Chaber, L. (2007). *The Thing Inside my Head: A Family's Journey Through Mental Illness.* Essex, U.K.: Chipmunkapublishing.

Charbit, A. (2011). *A Life Lived Ridiculously.* Snellville, GA: Firefly Publishing & Entertainment.

Claypole-White, B. (2012). *The Unfinished Garden.* Buffalo, NY: Harlequin.

Colas, E. (1999). *Just Checking: Scenes From the Life of an Obsessive-Compulsive.* New York: Washington Square Press.

Curtis, V. (2010). *Zelah Green: Who Says I'm a Freak?.* London: Egmont.

Deane, R. (2005). *Washing My Life Away: Surviving Obsessive Compulsive Disorder.* London: Jessica Kingsley Publishers.

Fadem, R. (2003). *Memoirs of a Born Shlepper: Never Give OCD a Third Thought.* New York: Shleppedicke Press.

Foust, T. (2011). *Nowhere Near Normal: A Memoir of OCD.* New York: Gallery Books.

Frederique (2012). *No ocd: One Family's Journey Through Obsessive Compulsive Disorder.* Bloomington, IN: iUniverse.

Gander, B. (2009). *OCD & Me.* Petersfield: Gander Publications.

Gleason, K. (2007). *Obsessed...A Tale of OCD, Knitting, and Inappropriate Men.* LuLu.

Guis, M. (2006). *Living with Severe OCD.* Bothwell, WA: Book Publishers Network.

Hartman, R. (2012). *Life in Mental Chains.* Louisville, KY: Turquoise Morning.

Hesser, T. (1999). *Kissing Doorknobs.* New York: Laurel Leaf.

Jordan, T. (2010). *Addition.* Salem, OR: Polebridge Press.

Kant, J. (2008). *The Thought That Counts.* Oxford: University Press.

Kaufman, A. (2011). *Oxford Messed Up: A Novel.* Chicago: Grant Place Press.

Keller, J. (2012). *I Hardly Ever Wash My Hands.* St. Paul: Paragon House.

Limburg, J. (2010). *The Woman Who Thought Too Much.* London: Atlantic Books.

Maloney, B. (2009). *Saving Sammy: Curing the Boy Who Caught OCD.* New York: Crown Publishers.

Mukherjee, S. (2011). *A Life Interrupted.* Bloomington, IN: Xlibris Corporation.

Murphy, T. (2009). *Life in Rewind: The Story of a Young Man Who Persevered Over OCD and the Harvard Doctor Who Broke All the Rules to Help Him.* New York: William Morrow.

Osborn, I. (1999). *Tormenting Thoughts and Rituals: The Hidden Epidemic of Obsessive-Compulsive Disorder.* New York: Dell.

Pascaris, P. (2007). *Desert Lily.* Bloomington, IN: iUniverse, Inc.

Patterson, J, and Friedman, H. (2008). *Against Medical Advice.* New York: Grand Central Publishing.

Pendred, V., ed. (2010). *Checkmates: A Collection of Fiction, Poetry, and Artwork About Obsessive-Compulsive Disorder, by People with OCD.* Conditional Publications.

Pope, H., Phillips, K., and Olivardia, R. (2000). *The Adonis Complex: How to Identify, Treat, and Prevent Body Obsession in Men and Boys.* New York: Simon and Schuster.

Radano, G. (2007). *Contaminated: My Journey Out of Obsessive Compulsive Disorder.* Scarsdale, NY: Bar-Le-Duc Books.

Rapoport, J. (1989). *The Boy Who Couldn't Stop Washing.* New York: Penguin Books.

Schwartz, J. (1996). *Brain Lock.* New York: Harper Perennial.

Schwartz, J. (2002). *The Mind and The Brain.* New York: Harper Perennial.

Shy, S. (2009). *It'll be Okay.* Bloomington, IN: Author House.

Summers, M. (1999). *Everything in its Place: My Trials and Triumphs with Obsessive Compulsive Disorder.* New York: Jeremy P. Tarcher/Putnam.

Traig, J. (2007). *Devil in the Details: Scenes From an Obsessive Girlhood.* New York: Back Bay Books.

Weg, A. (2011). *OCD Treatment Through Storytelling.* Oxford: University Press.

Wells, J. (2006). *Touch and Go Joe.* London: Jessica Kingsley Publishers.

White, D. (2007). *Overcoming OCD and Depression: My Personal Journey and Recovery.* Morgantown, PA: Masthof Press.

Wortmann, F. *(2012). Triggered: A Memoir of Obsessive-Compulsive Disorder.* New York: Thomas Dunne Books.

CPSIA information can be obtained at www.ICGtesting.com
Printed in the USA
LVOW10s0124190813

348450LV00002B/2/P